CREEK INDIAN MEDICINE WAYS

The Enduring Power of Mvskoke Religion

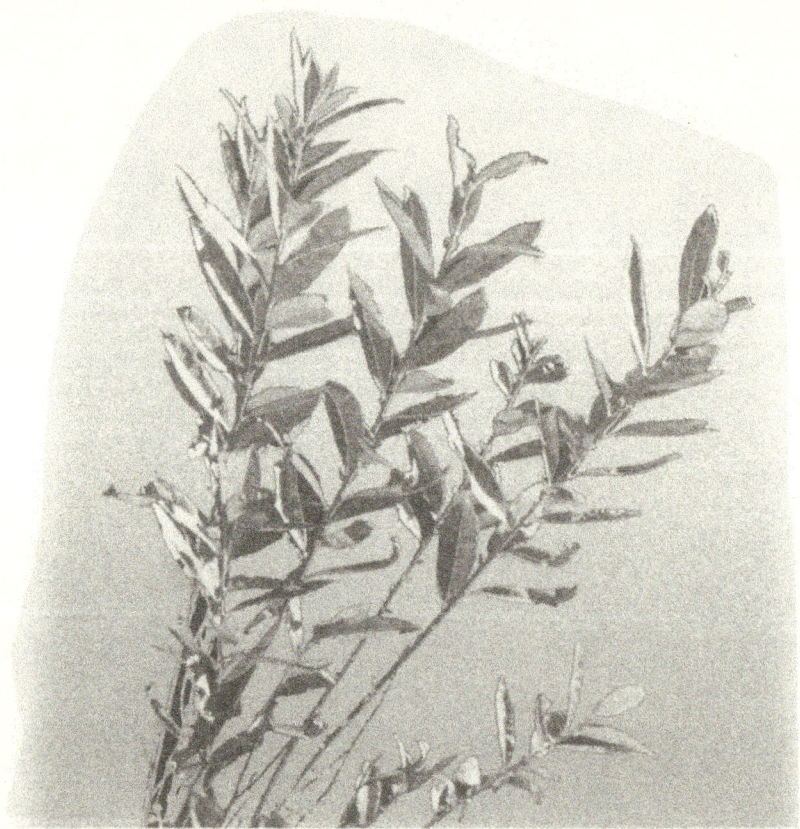

CREEK INDIAN MEDICINE WAYS

The Enduring Power of Mvskoke Religion

DAVID LEWIS JR.

ANN T. JORDAN

UNIVERSITY OF NEW MEXICO PRESS

ALBUQUERQUE

13 12 11 10 09 08   1 2 3 4 5 6

LIBRARY OF CONGRESS CATALOGING-IN-PUBLICATION DATA

Lewis, David, Jr., 1933–
Creek Indian medicine ways : the enduring power of Mvskoke religion /
David Lewis, Jr. and Ann T. Jordan. — 1st ed.
p.   cm.
ISBN 0-8263-2367-7
1. Creek Indians—Medicine. 2. Creek Indians—Religion.
I. Jordan, Ann T., 1946– II. Title.
E99.C9 L49 2002
615.8'2'089973—dc21
2001005455

DESIGN: MINA YAMASHITA

CONTENTS

PROLOGUE
David Lewis, Jr.

These are words my dad, David Lewis, Sr., said to me. The Grandpa he talks about is his grandfather, Jackson Lewis. The story his grandpa told him is about the removal. These words from my dad explain why we are losing our medicine culture.

"Sit right here. I'm going to tell you the story that my grandpa told to me as a young boy. These things I tell you, you must never forget. I'm telling you the same thing I was told, not to forget. Now I'm telling you. You don't forget. These things I'm telling you, not everybody knows these things. The Creator gave us these sacred words. These things that we have were left with us. Someday, it will be lost; you will see. You will see it being lost.

"This is what Grandpa told me:

"'They brought the people to the new land. There was death, hardship and heartache. They saw that as they were coming. The Indian people, the medicine people who were selected, they got angry. They were paying the white people back. The secret words were left with us. They made medicine that was not right. The medicine people called a meeting. I was with them.'

"The medicine people were the ones to carry on. They said you had to know that selected person, that you will know that he would not break the sacred words, that he will always be in good standing. It is going to be strict in selecting. This was what they were telling Grandpa when they were gathered there. If you can't find a replacement, when your days are ended, you will take with you all these words that were left with you.

"This is the instruction that was given out. This is what Grandpa told me. You are very young. You may wonder, 'Why are you telling me this?' The medicine people that were supposed to carry on are getting less. This is what I see now. Everything has a start. There is also an ending. What I see now. The things that will be lost are upon us now. I see this. That is why I am talking to you. Grandpa, he was talking to me. Grandpa told me that story."

PREFACE

This book is the result of a collaboration between a full-blood Mvskoke (Creek) medicine man (Lewis) and a Euro-American anthropologist (Jordan). To clarify our respective roles in the project, we present joint opening observations in the third person, followed by personal statements explaining our reasons for undertaking the work.

David Lewis is a member of the Bird Clan and of Hickory Ground Tribal Town in northeastern Oklahoma. He is the only living, initiated Mvskoke medicine person and here he puts in writing the information he thinks is important for the Mvskoke people to know about their medicine tradition. This information has been passed down orally through generations of initiated medicine people and much of it would be unknown even to Mvskoke people not initiated as medicine people. Ann Jordan provides a context for Lewis's information by explaining the written history of the Mvskoke, their religion and medicine, and the history of Lewis's extraordinary medicine family. His family is well documented in the written record. His great grandfather, a renowned medicine man, was the source of much information on Mvskoke religion collected by anthropologists in the early twentieth century.

Two introductory chapters on history, written primarily by Jordan, acquaint the reader with the Mvskoke people, their history and culture, and with Lewis's family. The first of these chapters describes the history of the Mvskoke people, as it is found in the written record, to provide an understanding of the five centuries of struggle that the Mvskoke people have endured to keep their culture and way of life. The Mvskoke medicine way, which is documented from the earliest written records of the *Mvskokvlke*, continues today. The second chapter relates the history of Lewis's well-known medicine family, including his own brief personal account but consisting largely of background found in the written record on the individuals mentioned in his narrative. It also explains the family's previous contribution to the anthropological understanding of Mvskoke culture and religion. Much of what is already known about Mvskoke religion was provided by Jackson Lewis, David Lewis's great grandfather, to John Swanton, a well-known ethnographer with the Bureau of American Ethnology in 1910. David Lewis's contribution in this book is of particular significance to anthropologists, historians, and other students of Mvskoke culture and history because it continues the work of Swanton and Jackson Lewis by describing Jackson Lewis's medicine knowledge as practiced almost a century after his death.

The heart of the book consists of Lewis's description of the living medicine tradition. His medicine training was conducted in the Mvskoke language, which is his primary language; several sections of the text, notably the teaching of his father in the prologue and "The Story" (chapter 6), are direct translations from Mvskoke. Lewis begins with an explanation of kinds of medicine people (chapter 3). It is important to distinguish these in order to understand much of what follows. There are three types of medicine people, all of whom are referred to as *heles-hayv* (medicine maker). The first one Lewis discusses is the main medicine person who is initiated and taught full knowledge of medicine for both good and bad purposes. Lewis is this type of medicine person. A main medicine person passes his or her knowledge on to only one individual through a training process. Thus for each person in this category, there is a single replacement. These individuals are the only ones with the power to see the visions for new cures. The second type of medicine person is the "carrier." A carrier is selected by a main medicine person to learn a selected set of cures but is not given the full knowledge or fully initiated, nor will he or she see visions of new cures. Such a person is selected to "carry" the words of some of the cures known by a main medicine person. A carrier could also train another carrier sharing that knowledge. The third type is the specialist, the ceremonial ground medicine person. This individual makes medicine for the ceremonial ground and for the Mvskoke traditional ceremonies held on that ground. All of these types of medicine people may be powerful and well respected.

In chapter 4, Lewis describes his own selection, training, and initiation as a main *heles-hayv*. His detailed description reveals the rigor, complexity, and comprehensiveness of Mvskoke medicine. This training is little known by other Mvskoke, for it was never discussed openly. It is described in print for the first time here. In chapter 5 Lewis tells of growing up in a family of well-known medicine people. Together, these two chapters provide valuable insights into the Mvskoke world. Storytelling is a well developed art among the Mvskoke, and these chapters show Lewis's ability in this important art while, at the same time, describing a sacred tradition.

Lewis feels that "The Story" (chapter 6) is the most significant information he can share with his people. This sacred narrative explains the origin of the Mvskoke medicine way, giving the origin of medicine plants, explaining the powers that medicine people would have, and presenting the rules they must follow. This rendering contains only parts of the story because it is too sacred for Lewis to reveal in its entirety. The rest of Lewis's chapters on medicine are based on the knowledge gained from the story.

The native plants in northeastern Oklahoma are well-known to Lewis and have traditional importance. He lists some of these plants and their traditional medicine uses in chapter 7. In Mvskoke medicine, the plant alone cannot bring about a cure. It must be combined with a sacred chant. No chants are revealed in this book. They are too sacred; to commit them to writing would be extremely sacrilegious.

The requirements of the medicine life are presented in chapter 8. A medicine person must not only know the plants and the chants, but must also keep himself or herself spiritually strong. Lewis explains this and then discusses a series of cures, indicating how he decides what to use to cure a person and describing the process of treating a patient. In chapter 9 he describes three ceremonies he might be called upon to perform. The first, a Blessing Ceremony, he performed at the old Creek Council House in Okmulgee, Oklahoma. The second, Doctoring a House, he has conducted numerous times. The third, the Reburial Ceremony, he has never been called upon to perform. This ceremony would be used to move a grave from one location to another. As a result of the Native American Graves Protection and Repatriation Act of 1990, many American Indian tribes are bringing home skeletal remains, grave goods, and ceremonial objects from museums and other public places in which they have been stored for a century or more. In addition to its use in moving a grave, this Reburial Ceremony could be used to bring home the remains of Mvskoke burials, which are housed in museums. In the concluding chapter Lewis offers his opinions about medicine, both the sacred and the scientific, and about his sacred world.

In the appendices, Jordan provides further documentation explaining how Lewis's information fits into the existing record on Mvskoke history, culture, and medicine. As noted, the Lewis family already holds an important place in the documentation of Mvskoke medicine. The appendices contextualize Lewis's contribution within that documentation and the larger written record while demonstrating how the interpretations of Mvskoke religion through the centuries reflect the agendas and worldviews of their authors. Also, when Lewis's words are placed in the context of the previous written record on the Mvskoke, one sees how the rich and multilayered Mvskoke culture has endured and changed over the centuries.

Throughout this work Mvskoke words are employed. Translations for these appear in the text and again in the glossary. While the Mvskoke are typically known both in the written record and in common English usage as the Creek, Lewis determined that they should be referred to by the name *Mvskoke* in this book. The name *Creek* was originally used by the English to refer to the inhabitants along Ochesee Creek (the upper Ocmulgee River) and later expanded to refer to the indigenous inhabitants of the Southeast who were not Cherokee, Chickasaw, or Choctaw. Mvskoke is the name used to refer to the Creeks if one is speaking the Mvskoke language, although the word is probably not a Muskogean word, but rather a Shawnee word originally used by the Shawnee to refer to the Mvskoke in the Southeast and later adopted by the Mvskoke themselves.[1] Lewis also determined that in this book words in his language should be spelled using the Mvskoke alphabet. Thus, the name is spelled *Mvskoke* rather than *Muscogee*. This alphabet was used in the *English and Muskokee Dictionary* published by R. M. Loughridge, a Presbyterian missionary who began work among the Mvskoke in 1842, and David M. Hodge, a Mvskoke interpreter and elder. The alphabet continues in use today and is used in *A Dictionary of Creek/Muskogee* published by Jack Martin and Margaret Mauldin in 2000. It is used in all spellings of Mvskoke words in this text with the exception of names of towns and tribal grounds for which the English spellings are more commonly used. The modern political entity that is the tribal nation is officially designated the Muscogee (Creek) Nation and is so named in this text. *Muskogee* is used to designate the language as well as the city in Oklahoma. Generally, *Indian* or *American Indian* is used to refer to Native Americans and *white* or *Euro-Americans* to refer to that non-Mvskoke body.

Many individuals and organizations have helped the authors during this project. Particular thanks go to the following: The University of North Texas provided financial assistance. Jack Martin and Margaret Mauldin gave advice on the spelling of Mvskoke words. Sally Antrobus, Brooke Fugit, and Floyce Alexander provided valuable editorial assistance. Durwood Ball, Evelyn Schlatter, and David Holtby at the University of New Mexico Press were sensitive shepherds of the project. The anonymous reviewers provided invaluable suggestions for improvement. The authors, however, assume sole responsibility for any errors in the work.

THE MEDICINE MAN'S VOICE
David Lewis, Jr.

I know that I'm the only living, true medicine man left who has actually been initiated. It is nothing to brag about; it makes me sad. We have a lot of carriers (uninitiated medicine people) who practice our medicine and they are very strong people, but they do not know the history of the origin of our medicine. The tribe has ceremonial grounds and they use these red roots all through the summer and the other medicine people use the red roots, but they don't know the history of where red roots came from. The history of our medicine is only taught to the initiated medicine people. I haven't found a replacement to initiate to carry on this medicine culture. There is an old story that says you will be given time to find one. Maybe that is why the medicine people lived to be old people; they put off finding a replacement. But you just can't find a candidate as easy as it sounds because the selection process is so strict. I don't think I will ever find one.

The prologue of this book is what my dad said to me. He was explaining what was told to him by his grandpa, Jackson Lewis. He was talking about the removal in the 1830s when the Mvskoke were forced to move from Alabama and Georgia to Indian Territory. It explains why we are losing our medicine culture. There was a lot of death when they were coming during the removal. A lot of the medicine people, their loved ones died on the way. These were very powerful medicine people and they got very angry and they wanted to get back at the white people. The only way they knew how to do it was to make bad medicine with the material things that would be buried with their loved ones. Medicine was made and those belongings were treated and buried with their loved ones so that any time anybody ever dug into the graves of their loved ones, it would release the bad that they did. They knew that the Indian people would never fool with their graves, but only the whites would. So in order to get back at the white people, the bad medicine was made. What they were doing was very destructive. It would kill. They were that powerful and that wasn't to be done. It started getting out of hand.

That is why the wise people, the main medicine people, gathered all the medicine people. This is the meeting my great grandfather, Jackson, was telling my dad about. From that day on, from that meeting, they started the selection process that we still use to decide which child will be a medicine person. They gave the instruction that you will know your replacement; the child will be tested. Now they had to know: will this child ever misuse this medicine that I'm going to give to him? I'll give him good, I will also give him bad medicine. Is he or she going to misuse this medicine down the future, sixty years from now?

As a medicine person, you walk a fine line. If you misuse the medicine, you can never do only good anymore. You have broken your tradition, your culture of your learning. Before the removal, they were good, caring people, but they broke the tradition and they went the wrong way. In order for them not to lose any more of what they were doing, they made a strict rule from there on out: you will select a replacement who will not ever break the tradition of your culture; it will always be kept sacred. If you do not find your replacement, then you will take the medicine knowledge to your grave.

And that was the beginning of losing our medicine culture, back then in the removal, because of what they did to get back at the white people. The selection process was so strong and strict that it is hard to find a replacement. They always talked about the removal which was a very sad thing that happened. But the way I look at it, probably the saddest part was the beginning of losing our medicine culture because of what took place. That's more important to me.

It reminds me of the last gathering of the eight most powerful, initiated, Mvskoke people that I witnessed when I was a child. The medicine people were very secret. You couldn't even be around them when they were talking about medicine if you weren't one of the initiated medicine people. It wasn't allowed; you would be asked to leave. The medicine people didn't only talk about their technique, they would prophesy about what would be today. The plants that they had been using that were plentiful, they said that in your time they will be hard to get. They were talking about me, because I remember sitting on their laps and they said, "You will see in your time that medicines that are plentiful today will be scarce." They said, "We are losing our sacred plants in the name of progress. A lot of the plants will be destroyed." So I see these things that are coming to pass and someday our medicine will be very weak. There will be no one around to pass these ways down to. It will no longer be here. We will only have carriers. I know it is coming. Dad and I knew it. My grandmother knew it. She said that she didn't want to be here when we lose this. But she said, "You'll be here. You will be here and see the origin of our medicine culture come to an end. It will be gone." I think she meant that I would probably be the last person who knows the history of our medicine culture and it will be taken with me upon my death.

My great grandfather, Jackson Lewis, seemed to know that Dad was going to write about our medicine culture because he told him: "You are very talented. I believe that you will someday talk about it." Just like Dad always said to me, "I know you are going to talk about it." Jackson Lewis kind of thought that Dad would, but Dad didn't talk about it. I thought about it for years and years from way back. Dad and I talked about it, and he said, "Son, I know someday you are going to talk about it, but be careful of what you give out, because it's not for everybody. It is only to pass down to the one who will replace you to know this history of this, our sacred ways." Dad wouldn't talk about it. There was no way they could ever talk to my grandmother about it. I thought about it for so long, though, that I know what I want to say and I know what part I'm going to leave out. There are no songs or sacred words in what we write in this book like we saw in other books because I do not believe in that. It is not given out that way. What we are writing about here was passed down to me in my family. This is only how the Lewis and Jacob family does it. Other medicine people use different roots and the words they use are different from ours. In our family the sacred words are built around animals, nature, and human beings. I don't know how the others were trained in other families; this is the way I was trained.

With that in mind, I just thought it was time I shared some of these things with my people. There is no one else around to talk about this. Today we have forty-eight thousand citizens of the Muscogee (Creek) Nation and yet we have less than two thousand full-bloods. I know firsthand who the medicine people are. I grew up around them and their families. My family took care of the families whose offspring are practicing medicine now. Some of them making medicine now were little kids and some were not even born. I sat with them when their families asked my family questions. Anyone who is initiated would never ask anyone else how to make a medicine because they would have all the knowledge and power they needed. When people come around asking, that is the telltale sign they are not initiated. The gathering of the last eight that I have talked about; now those were initiated people. Anybody who was not initiated could not have sat with them. If I had not already been initiated, I would not have been allowed to sit with them that fall. That was in the early 1940s and there were only eight left. By the 1950s, only about three of them were left. In 1955, my grandmother died and in 1985 my dad died. People making medicine now, most of them are not even sixty yet; so, most of them were not even born. The medicine people we have today, I knew their parents and those were the people who were asking questions about how to make medicine from my family and they would never have been doing that if they were initiated.

After the medicine is gone, it's gone. But if it's in written form, maybe someday the Mvskoke people will take this book off the shelf and say, "We had some powerful people at one time. We missed out on a lot of things. We should have been listening." Today nobody listens because they think it is going to be here forever. And it is not going to be and I know it and I see it coming. A lot of these things have never been brought out. They have no idea and I just wanted to share some of these with my own people.

The most important thing, I guess, is keeping the whole thing sacred. You have to live this every day, seven days a week, twenty-four hours a day to make sure you don't get caught not being prepared. You are liable to get called anytime. So you have to be prepared at a minute's notice. That is how dedicated a person is supposed to be and it's not happening and I know it and I see it all the time. I know what I have and what to do. I act crazy sometimes, but when you get down to the medicine, I am very serious. It is hard; it is a rough road. There is nothing easy about this. We lose a lot of sleep, travel long ways. You go look for roots when it's raining. It doesn't make any difference, you have got to go when you need certain medicines that have to be freshly dug. The people think there's plenty of medicine out there, or like I went out and bought some, which I would never do. They don't see what is behind the scenes, what you have to go through just to be prepared for them. That is the hard part, they have no idea what a medicine person has to go through to take care of our people.

I'm glad that we wrote this book. It means a lot to me. If we can just show the remaining Mvskoke people that we had some powerful medicine people out there among us at one time, I will be satisfied. In somebody's family once lived a medicine person who was a powerful person and it is gone. That is something that cannot be picked up and carried on because they took it with them. That is one reason we are losing it, and I didn't want to just lose it completely without ever sharing it with somebody, with our people, what the medicine is all about. So I decided that I wanted to tell the beginning, how we got these things and why it is so sacred. If it's written down, then if they are interested enough about our history of our medicine people, maybe they'll search back and they may remember their grandparents, what they used to do, and see all the good things that we have today that may not be here tomorrow.

THE ANTHROPOLOGIST'S VOICE
Ann T. Jordan

As an anthropologist involved in a collaborative project with a practicing Mvskoke medicine person, I have found the writing of this book to be a journey of discovery into both the traditional Mvskoke medicine world of my coauthor and the traditional academic world of my own profession. I have learned significantly about both. The book is written with two agendas: David Lewis's agenda, as described in his preface, is to write down for the Mvskoke people some of the knowledge about traditional medicine ways that is unknown to them; my agenda is to contribute to the anthropological and historical knowledge of Mvskoke culture and to our understanding of the ways in which anthropologists and other non-Mvskoke represent that culture. David Lewis's audience is the Mvskoke community of which he is a member. My audience is the academic community of which I am a member. We both additionally hope that the book is of interest to general readers outside our particular fields of influence.

I thought long and hard about the appropriate way to represent David Lewis's story and my related commentary in written form. I appreciate the insights of those anthropologists who stress that traditionally the ethnographer's voice, though purposely hidden, has been the dominant controller and shaper of works of ethnography. I also appreciate the critique of American Indian scholars who suggest that non-Indian researchers frequently misrepresent Indian societies. Consequently, I wish to describe in detail the process of writing this book and the reasons for the particular form it takes.

The content was determined entirely by David Lewis. From the beginning we had an agreement that he would determine the content and that I would not press him for information he chose not to reveal. In the course of the research, I asked him many questions. However, when he told me my question referred to an area about which he did not wish to speak, the question was not pursued. This agreement was to protect the sacred nature of the information he was sharing. The chapter divisions were developed by the two of us. The text belonging to David Lewis was taken from narrative that he tape recorded or wrote out. I then transcribed the tapes, edited the tapes and written sections, and returned them to him for further editing. My coauthor is a scrupulous editor. Due to the sacred nature of this material and its extreme importance to him, he read and reread the manuscript many times. We agreed that the book would take a rather traditional form in which David Lewis's information is presented in a first-person narrative and my comments, which place his work in the context of the written anthropological and historical tradition, are presented in introductory chapters and appendices.

Aside from the difference in the reading populations we wish to serve and the agendas we bring to the project, I was struck by the difference in our commitments to oral and written tradition. David Lewis is providing information that has been passed down orally and is being written down for the first time. His telling of the information in the first person, as it personally affected him, was so compelling that it would have seemed a violation to alter the form of the story. Consequently, it is presented as he spoke and wrote it. I did not wish to disturb the flow of his story by interjecting my academic commentary. Thus I made the decision to place my commentary in separate chapters and as appendices. Further, I felt that my contribution was not best represented in a first-person narrative. This book is about David Lewis's story, not mine. My primary contribution is to place his story in the context of other written accounts of Mvskoke religion and culture and to assist in bringing his story into the written tradition. Consequently, it made sense to me to place my comments, other than this introductory section, in the third person. Even in my third-person comments, however, my enthusiasm for first-person Mvskoke narrative is made obvious by the number of excerpts from the Indian Pioneer Papers scattered throughout my portion of the text. These materials collected in the 1930s provide rich accounts by Mvskoke individuals, most of which have not previously been easily accessible in print.

To clarify my position further, I would like to describe some of my experiences, emotions, and perspectives involving this project. The first is a lesson I learned about the fragility of professional truth. Even with the careful attention to accuracy with which I approached this project, I discovered that accuracy was not within my professional control; I have come to understand the ease with which ethnographers err in reporting "the facts." I learned this lesson through the following experience. David Lewis said to me on more than one occasion, "You and I live in two different worlds and I can come into your world but you can't come into mine." I would nod, "yes," thinking, "of course this is true." I could clearly see that he lives in an Indian world full of Indian family and friends, living according to his traditional Mvskoke values and working for his tribe both as a medicine man and as a member of the tribal council. I live in a white world of family and friends, working in a culturally white, academic institution. Lewis has spent his entire life negotiating between his world and the white world and is adept at maneuvering through both. I have not been in the position of being forced to negotiate between two cultural systems throughout my lifetime. Even though familiar with the Indian world, I do not have the skills to understand and negotiate that world in the way that he has the skills to understand and negotiate the white one. Having made the comment about the two separate worlds to me several times, David Lewis said nothing to change my understanding of his comment. Eventually, however, he taught me a valuable professional lesson. This is the story he told.

When the time comes for me to go into the woods to fast for four days I've already made up my mind what years of my life I want to see. I go to the sacred ground or square and use the medicine I have prepared for this occasion. After I have finished all the things I was taught to do, I usually lean back and close my eyes and go back in time. I have gone back to the day I was being born. I have watched my mom push me out into this world as my grandmother received or delivered me and my dad standing close by their side with the medicine in his hand that was to be used on me. I watched as they gave me some medicine to drink and washed me down with another type of medicine to work on my motor system.

I have gone back to the time I began to walk. This was a time of training in how to identify the medicine plants you are going to use the rest of your life for your people. You learn the type of flower and color of certain plants and whether they grow tall or stay close to the ground. You learn the type of bark on the tree and the shape of the leaves and their colors. I have watched myself as my grandmother or dad gave me a medicine root and had me smell and bite into the root so I would know what it tasted like. I have gone back to the days of initiations many times, for what reason I still don't know. It could be the energy or power of the unknown that I witness on that day. I have gone back to the time when as a little boy I sat on my grandmother's lap as she recited the medicine words that some day I would follow the footsteps of our great people who have gone before.

The highlight of these fasts in my life is the encouragement of my grandmother or dad and other medicine people, their encouragement to keep myself strong, to sweat and wash the sacred words and purify my body so I would always be ready to do what is asked of me for our people. It is always hard to let go of my grandmother and dad's voices and their presence. It wants to make you cry, but I was taught to never cry for medicine people not even in death, which I went through twice. I'm always thankful I had a short visit with my loved ones.

This story was a lesson for the anthropologist, although, not being accustomed to learning through stories, I had to have it spelled out for me before I understood. David Lewis went on to explain.

So what I meant when I said we live in two worlds and I can come into yours but you can't step over into mine was these two realities. You cannot come into the reality of the medicine people. It is different from the reality of this world. And you will never know it. You will never know what that change of energy is like. But you didn't understand what I meant before. I didn't give you enough information to understand what I meant. You tried to figure out what I meant with what knowledge you had and you didn't know about this other world of mine. I am in your world but I can also live in my world that no person can come into.

I finally realized that Lewis was explaining why I was not getting it right and, by extension, why anthropologists so often do not get it right. Our "informants" are in control of the knowledge we gain. They can choose to share, or choose to leave us with misunderstandings or no understandings. No amount of participant observation would have prevented my misunderstanding as I would never have been able to witness the sacred event he described. No matter how much time we spend with them, we anthropologists who are outsiders do not live in the worlds of the people we "study." Without those lived experiences, we do not know the right questions to ask. I took it for granted that I understood what Lewis meant when he spoke of our two worlds. He knew I was misunderstanding, but chose not to correct my misunderstanding. When he finally did so, I gained some professional humility and valuable insight.

This project was rewarding in other ways as well. Years ago, as an anthropology graduate student particularly interested in American Indian cultures, I spent many an hour in the library stacks poring over old volumes of the Bureau of American Ethnology bulletins and annual reports. They seemed to me then and still seem now to be a treasure trove of ethnographic information. To me, these books were artifacts out of the past; their pages were yellow, brittle, and dusty. The world they described seemed remote and floating in timelessness. Knowing many American Indians at the time, I realized that American Indian cultures had flourished and continued as vibrant, living traditions, but those living communities did not, for me, seem connected to the old volumes published by the BAE.

They did not seem connected, that is, until years later when I met David Lewis. At that meeting, I learned of his role as a medicine person, but it was some time before I discovered his connection to those dusty volumes in the library of my graduate-school days. Jackson Lewis, David Lewis's great grandfather, was one of John Swanton's primary informants on Mvskoke religion. John Swanton's BAE publications on the Mvskoke (1922, 1928a, 1928b, 1931, 1946) remain a primary source of information on the tribe. In Swanton's *Religious Beliefs and Medical Practices of the Creek Indians*, Jackson Lewis is referenced by name seventy-six times in the 193 pages of text (1928b). David Lewis's medicine knowledge was learned from his father and his mother's mother, both initiated medicine people. His father learned medical knowledge directly from Jackson Lewis, Swanton's informant. Thus David Lewis is the direct recipient of Jackson Lewis's medicine knowledge through a single intermediary, David Lewis's father (David Lewis, Sr.).

Upon realizing this, I suddenly felt as if those dusty volumes in the library basement had sprung off the shelves and come to life. The pages now held real people, whom I almost felt I knew. In addition, I learned that David Lewis was unaware that his great grandfather was even mentioned in any anthropological accounts of the tribe and certainly unaware of his prominence in these classic works on the Mvskoke. It was a great pleasure and honor for me to be able to provide him copies of these volumes holding his great grandfather's words. The discovery also led me into an archival search into the history of Lewis's family and the interesting intertwining of written and oral traditions. The resulting rendering of our joint work therefore involves an interplay of several voices besides our own, including those of Lewis's forebears and a series of ethnographers.

I feel that anthropologists have a responsibility to give back to the people with whom they work in an exchange that is mutually beneficial. Providing the Lewis family with copies of Swanton's work was one way in which I was able to do that. Writing a collaborative book is another. In this book David Lewis and I intend to serve both our audiences and both our agendas. I provide the researcher's anthropological and historical context. He provides the story.

Introduction

THE HISTORICAL CONTEXT

Chapter One

HISTORY OF THE MVSKOKE

The Mvskoke today are the proud members of vibrant cultures whose survival of five centuries of contact is testimony to the strength of the people and their way of life. Here, the story of those five centuries is told in order to place today's Mvskoke world and its living, traditional religion in context.

Prior to the nineteenth century, it was almost impossible to learn about Mvskoke history from the Mvskoke point of view if one based that history on the written record. The early record consists of archaeological findings. The first written sources were authored almost exclusively by European and Euro-American explorers, missionaries, Indian agents, and traders, whose perspectives are centered in their own cultures. The remainder of the record is found, for the most part, in legal documents like treaties, government reports, court cases, and census counts. In the last century, however, the Mvskoke point of view appears frequently in the written record. Much of this information is oral tradition that has been committed to written form in interviews with and stories told by Mvskoke people about their past or in written records pertaining to the sovereign entity, now known as the Muscogee (Creek) Nation.

MVSKOKE ORIGINS AND THE ARCHAEOLOGICAL RECORD

At a certain time, the Earth opened in the West, where its mouth is. The earth opened and the Cussitaws came out of its mouth, and settled near by. But the earth became angry and ate up their children; therefore they moved further west. A part of them, however, turned back, and came again to the same place where they had been, and settled there. The greater number remained behind, because they thought it best to do so. Their children, nevertheless, were eaten by the Earth, so that, full of dissatisfaction, they journeyed toward the sunrise.[1]

This is the earliest written account of the origins of the Mvskoke people. It was presented by Tchikilli, a Mvskoke leader, in a speech given at Savannah in 1735. Tchikilli presented Governor Oglethorpe of the English colony of Georgia with a buffalo skin on which was depicted this account of the origins of his people. He explained how the Cusseta group of Mvskoke traveled east and crossed many rivers and mountains. Along the way they were joined by and met other groups who would eventually become part of the Mvskoke Confederacy. They also obtained their sacred fire and sacred plants such as *mēkko-hoyvnēcv* (*Salix humilis* Marsh). Thus, this first written account by a Mvskoke individual of origins of the Mvskoke people also includes important information about religious practices.

According to the archaeological record, prior to European contact the Mvskoke lived in present-day Georgia and Alabama as a part of what is termed the Mississippian culture, dating from 800 A.D. to 1500 A.D. As members of this prehistoric culture, the Mvskoke lived in towns of two to three thousand. The most prominent features of these towns still visible today are earth mounds, sometimes forty to fifty feet tall, which probably supported ceremonial structures. Archaeologists surmise that the Mississippian culture had a religious and political structure in which towns were either autonomous or members of a larger political chiefdom or confederacy. The people created beautiful artwork of unique design in stone and shell as well as weapons, copper ornaments, and wooden statues. Most of these works of art would have been steeped in religious significance. The people were horticulturalists whose primary crop was maize. Ocmulgee National Monument near present-day Macon, Georgia, is an example of a Mississippian site that would have been inhabited by the ancestors of the Mvskoke.[2] During the fourteenth century, the Mississippian culture began to decline. The arrival of DeSoto in 1539 heralded its final demise. Warfare with the Europeans, combined with epidemics of the diseases they brought, caused overwhelming population loss. The Mississippian culture disappeared. The cultures that replaced it in the Southeast are those there today, primarily the Cherokee, Chickasaw, Choctaw, Seminole, and Mvskoke Creek.[3]

MVSKOKE LIFE IN THE SOUTHEAST, 1500–1700

For two centuries after those first contacts with European explorers, Mvskoke life was rich, full, and unhampered by Europeans. Some details of this life can be pieced together from accounts by later writers.[4] Like their Mississippian ancestors, the Mvskoke were horticulturalists. Maize was their staple food, supplemented by beans, melons, and squash. They fished with spears, harpoons, bows and arrows, and weirs and hunted for deer, bear, rabbit, squirrel, turkey, and other birds. Wild plants supplemented these foods. Women worked the fields with hoes and digging sticks. The people lived in towns or *tvlwv* located along a stream or a river. Within a town, each matrilocal family might have a compound of gardens, fields, and several buildings, including a summer and a winter house.[5] The center of the town included a ball court, a ceremonial ground, and a council house. Four houses situated one on each of four sides of the ceremonial ground were occupied during special occasions by the men of the town, who positioned themselves in the houses according to their various titles. The *mēkkvlke* (town chiefs) occupied one, the *tvstvnvke* (warriors) occupied a second, the *cēpvnvke* (youths) the third, and the *henehvlke* (assistants to the chief) a fourth.[6]

The *tvlwv* or towns were autonomous. There was no single government ruling all Mvskoke, although at times the *tvlwv* did form a loose alliance that came to be known as the Creek Confederacy. The *tvlwv* included speakers of nine distinct languages. Six of these—Muskogee, Alabama, Koasati, Hitchitee, Mikasuki, and Apalachee—are closely related and belong to the Muskogean linguistic group. Choctaw and Chickasaw, languages spoken by two of the other large southeastern tribes who were not part of this alliance or confederacy, are also languages in the Muskogean linguistic family. The confederacy additionally included the Natchez, the Yuchi, and the Shawnee. The Natchez language is distantly related to the Muskogean language family, and together the two comprise the Natchez Muskogean stock. The Yuchi and Shawnee languages are in no way related to the Muskogean family. Yuchi is probably of the Siouan linguistic family and Shawnee of the Algonquian linguistic family.[7]

Thus the *tvlwv* of the confederacy contained many linguistic and ethnic groups: (1) the Muskogee speakers who originally inhabited the towns of Coweta, Cusseta, Coosa, and Abihka; (2) the Hitchitee; (3) the Alabama, who earlier may have had their own confederacy incorporating the Koasatis, Tawasas, and Tuskegees and including several languages in the Muskogean family; (4) the Yuchis; (5) a small group of the Shawnee, whose culture and language retained Algonquian characteristics; and (6) the Natchez, who had been driven east from their homeland on the Mississippi by the French.[8]

Some towns were closely affiliated with others. If one became too large, groups might split off to form new towns, which would be allied with the original or "mother" town. All Mvskoke were members of matrilineal, exogamous clans, like Bird, Bear, Turkey, and Wind. These clans were further combined into groups. It is not clear what the function of the kinship groupings larger than the clan was. They may have represented larger exogamous units. What is clear is that it was always improper to marry within one's clan. Clans crosscut towns and clan obligations were strong. Thus the autonomous towns were linked together by the clan system. Specific sets of rules of behavior applied to members of one's own clan and other rules to other clans to which one was related, like the father's clan. A person visiting a distant town would expect members of his or her clan, if such was to be found in that town, to provide food and a place to stay. Clan kin were responsible for punishment, revenge, education, and marriage arrangements. Ceremonial responsibilities in a town were clan inherited. Additionally, towns were divided into two groups: white and red, representing peace and war respectively. Peace councils were conducted by the leaders of the white towns and war was a matter for leaders of the red ones. A red or white stick positioned at the town announced its position to outsiders. Towns were known to change from white to red and vice versa. Clans were also identified as either red or white, although a clan might be white in one town and red in another.[9]

Religion pervaded all of Mvskoke life. Several ceremonial activities are recorded in early accounts. The most important annual ceremony was the *posketv* (also spelled *poskita* or *boskita*, meaning "to fast"), called in English the Green Corn Ceremony, held in the summer. No one was allowed to eat new corn until after that ceremony. At that time all crimes that had occurred the previous year were forgiven, except for murder. The old fires were put out; a new one was lit at the ceremonial ground and from it all fires of the town were lit. This ceremony was described by many early chroniclers of Mvskoke life. It was an eight-day ceremony of extreme importance, involving the taking of medicine and special dances performed around the sacred, ceremonial fire. Another important ritual was a ceremony in which the men of the town would partake of a special drink or medicine made of yaupon or cassine leaves and called vsse by the Mvskoke and "black drink" by the Europeans. When guests arrived in the town, this ceremony of the taking of the black drink was conducted. In many towns this ceremony occurred daily. Most early chroniclers mention the black drink, and participated in the ceremony when they visited the towns. Every town had a *heles-hayv* (medicine maker) who was in charge of making medicine for all religious ceremonies of the town. Medicine made to cure ailments, to improve hunting, and for all other needs was made in a sacred manner by the *heles-hayv*. Ball games, called "the little brother of war," were conducted in the ball court in the center of town. These also were of a sacred nature and involved *heleswv* (medicine).

The exact nature of the deities in which the Mvskoke believed was unclear to the non-Mvskoke, but outsider chroniclers mention *Hesaketvmesē*, the Breath Holder or Master of Breath, as the most important of these. Other entities are also described, such as the tie snake, the horned snake, and the little people. The tie snake had originated from a transformed human being, and among its powers was the ability to catch an animal as large as a horse and drag it into the water. The horned snake was held in high esteem. Pieces of its horn had strong spiritual power. The little people were tiny people who could be seen by children and medicine people and who could aid medicine people.[10]

THE FUR TRADE YEARS, 1700–1800

When the English founded Charles Town in 1670, Mvskoke life changed forever. Early contact with the English focused on trade. The Mvskoke traded deerskins and Indian captives for guns, ammunition, cloth, tools, and weapons. Captives were sold as slaves in the Carolinas and the Caribbean. In the traditional Creek war pattern, male captives were killed and females and children adopted. With the advent of the slave trade, the Mvskoke simply traded these captives to the English. In 1715 the Yamasee tribe on the Carolina coast attacked and killed English settlers in retaliation for the capture of Yamasee for the slave trade. In order to prevent further unrest, the English government outlawed slave trade of Indian people. With only deerskins to trade, it is estimated Mvskoke hunters may have killed forty-five thousand to fifty thousand deer per year to this end.

During this time, the Mvskoke were successful in playing the English, Spanish, and French against one another and creating a balance that allowed them to maintain control of their lands and wealth. They negotiated with each of the European powers for alliances and trade. Given the relatively large population size and landholdings of the Mvskoke as well as the competition among the Europeans for strongholds in the New World, the Europeans saw alliances with the Mvskoke as improving their own strategic positions. A crucial factor in the Mvskoke maintaining this balance of power was their ability to trade skins for guns. Mvskoke adaptation to survival changed as they became commercial traders. While guns and ammunition were obviously crucial items to acquire through trade, other items like cloth were also important. The Mvskoke switched from skins to European material for clothing relatively early. During these early years of colonization, the Mvskoke were a powerful force. Mid-eighteenth-century estimates by various European and Georgian sources suggest that the population was ten to twelve thousand and the number of towns between fifty and eighty.[11]

A division developed between towns on the Chattahoochee and Flint rivers and those on the Alabama and its tributaries the Coosa and the Tallapoosa. The former were referred to as the "lower Mvskoke" and the latter as the "upper Mvskoke." The lower Mvskoke were physically located closer to European settlements and as a consequence intermarried more frequently with them and adopted more European customs. The upper Mvskoke, relatively isolated from such influences, retained greater adherence to traditional customs. More inhabitants of the upper towns were full-bloods. Red and white towns and clans occurred in both areas. The upper Mvskoke-lower Mvskoke division, however, became increasingly important in political events from the eighteenth century onward.

When the French and Indian War of 1763 resulted in the French retreating from the area, the Mvskoke were no longer able to play the three European powers against one another and were forced to deal primarily with the English. The American Revolution was to change the balance of power again. The Mvskoke, who remained neutral during the revolution, were later appalled to find that in the 1783 Treaty of Paris, much of their nation had been placed within the boundaries of a foreign power, the new United States. As sovereign nations, the Indians had not even been invited to the bargaining table.[12]

Alexander McGillivray was the first individual identified as Mvskoke to figure prominently in European and United States affairs. McGillivray was at most one-quarter Mvskoke as his father was the wealthy Scottish trader Lachlan McGillivray, and his mother was half Mvskoke and half French.[13] Alexander McGillivray owned plantations and slaves and controlled a large amount of the Mvskoke trading business. He was a silent partner in Panton, Leslie and Company, the largest deerskin trading company of the time, and was also a primary agent of the Spanish government with the Mvskoke. Announcing that he spoke for a confederacy of Mvskoke *tvlwv* and attempting to create a Mvskoke national council, McGillivray made treaties with Spain for weapons and with the United States to cede land in Georgia. The treaty with the United States included secret articles that greatly benefited McGillivray financially. Other *tvlwv* leaders were angry. Hopoithle Mico of Tallasee *tvlwv* and Eneah Mico of Cusseta *tvlwv* resisted and in fact had made treaties with the state of Georgia that preceded McGillivray's United States treaty. Pressure from the Georgia colonists, however, caused the leaders of the Mvskoke *tvlwv* to unite temporarily, and in 1790 Hopoithle Mico and McGillivray together signed a treaty with George Washington in New York.[14] LeClerc Milfort, a Frenchman and McGillivray's brother-in-law, stated that the treaty signing made McGillivray so unpopular among the Mvskoke that he feared for his life and left the Mvskoke lands.[15] McGillivray died shortly afterward.

The leadership of the new and still relatively weak United States was concerned about the Indians. In 1796 George Washington appointed Benjamin Hawkins as Indian agent. English by birth, Hawkins was a former North Carolina congressman. Hawkins's assignment was to acculturate the native populations so that they would behave like Euro-Americans; he could not understand the value in Mvskoke culture. He spent two decades among the Mvskoke trying to enforce the U.S. government policy of acculturation. To him the Mvskoke political system was anarchy and the economic system a communal disaster. He attempted to force the Mvskoke into a stronger central government, plow agriculture, hog and cattle raising, and town ownership of tribal land. This plan would, of course, free substantial Mvskoke lands for use by Euro-Americans. Already the differences between the upper Mvskoke, the more traditional, and the lower Mvskoke, the more acculturated, had appeared. Hawkins's efforts increased this division as the lower Mvskoke were more willing to take up Euro-American ways and accept his "civilization" program.[16]

THE RED STICK WAR AND
INCREASING LAND PRESSURE, 1800–1836

Mvskoke were becoming increasingly angry with Euro-American demands and influence on their traditional lifeways. In 1811 Tecumseh, a Shawnee prophet who predicted a return to the Indian way of life, visited Tuckabatchee *tvlwv*, which was a large and important upper Mvskoke town. Many Mvskoke accepted his prophecy. Soon afterward, his Mvskoke followers killed white settlers in Tennessee, and Agent Hawkins sent out a policing force of Mvskoke soldiers to avenge the murders. This began the Red Stick War of 1813–14. Red Stick, the Mvskoke symbol for war, was the name used to refer to Tecumseh's Mvskoke followers. At the same time the United States was fighting the War of 1812 and feared that the Mvskoke were allied with the British. The culmination of all this warfare for the Mvskoke came in the Battle of Horseshoe Bend, in which Jacksa Chula Harjo or "Old Mad Jackson" (known to non-Mvskoke as Andrew Jackson, Indian fighter and future president of the United States) defeated the Red Stick warriors of the upper Mvskoke.[17] At the Battle of Tohopeka alone, 800 Red Stick warriors died and 350 women and children were captured. It is thought that no later battle between American Indians and Euro-Americans caused as great a number of American Indian deaths. Estimates are that during this war two thousand to three thousand Mvskoke were killed and the fertile, productive towns of the upper Mvskoke were destroyed. A country of plenty was now a country of poverty and many suffered from famine. Benjamin Hawkins wrote of the destruction: "Look to the towns, not a living thing in them;

the inhabitants scattered through the woods, dying with hunger, or fed by Americans."[18] The backbone of the powerful Mvskoke Confederacy had been broken. With their population depleted and their economy in ruins, the Mvskoke were forced to surrender without payment twenty-five million acres of land in Alabama and Georgia in the Treaty of Fort Jackson in 1814. The 1810 census for Alabama listed 9,000 non-Indians; ten years later, the census listed 128,000 non-Indians. More than 100,000 whites had poured into the Mvskoke area in just ten years. The Mvskoke were losing control of their lands.[19]

The two decades between the Treaty of Fort Jackson and the final removal of the Mvskoke to Indian Territory was a time of torturous and complex political and economic struggles involving the Mvskoke, white intruders on their lands, the government of the United States, and the governments of the states of Georgia and Alabama. William McIntosh was to play an important role during this time period. The son of a Mvskoke mother and a Scottish father, McIntosh was a member of the Mvskoke town of Coweta and of the Wind Clan and was the leader of the Mvskoke forces who fought with Hawkins against the Red Stick faction. He was bribed by federal government officials and signed the Treaty of Indian Springs in 1824. By this time the Mvskoke had formed a national council and created a written code of law. The code included a law stating that should any Mvskoke individual sign a treaty giving up Mvskoke land, that individual would be put to death. McIntosh was executed in accordance with Mvskoke law. In this treaty McIntosh had ceded all Mvskoke lands in Georgia and two-thirds of the lands in Alabama.[20]

The Mvskoke refused to accept the fraudulent Treaty of Indian Springs. John Quincy Adams was now president. In 1826 a Mvskoke delegation led by Opothle Yoholo went to Washington. The United States pressured the delegation, telling them that if they did not agree to a new treaty, the United States would recognize the earlier, fraudulent McIntosh Treaty of Indian Springs and would force them to emigrate west of the Mississippi. The delegates agreed to the Treaty of Washington, in which the Mvskoke would cede the Georgia land but keep their Alabama lands. In the Treaty of Washington, the Mvskoke Confederacy would be paid roughly 250,000 dollars plus 20,000 dollars per year forever, and the United States acknowledged that the Treaty of Indian Springs was fraudulent. McIntosh's followers were allowed to emigrate to land set aside for them west of the Mississippi.[21]

Andrew Jackson became president in 1829 and in 1830 Congress passed the Indian Removal Act, which called for the removal of the Mvskoke to lands west of the Mississippi. The Mvskoke refused to sign a removal treaty. The whites in the state of Alabama were restless. In 1829 Alabamians had voted to make the Mvskoke people subject to Alabama law but not to make them citizens. Thus they could be punished for crimes and could be sued for legal infractions under Alabama law, but they could not testify in their own defense. Consequently the Mvskoke people suffered. Crimes against them were unpunished; fake deeds to their land could not be contested. The Euro-American citizens of Alabama had the right of legal harassment. Smallpox and starvation were taking their toll on the Alabama Mvskoke. In 1832 the Mvskoke sent a delegation to Washington to argue for reservations of land in the Southeast, equal legal rights for Mvskoke in Alabama, and restitution for the wrongs committed against them. A compromise was reached in the Treaty of 1832. The Mvskoke did receive reservations in the Southeast but had to sell their hunting lands. This meant they would need to change to market agriculture in order to survive economically. The United States was to protect Mvskoke property rights, but legal equality in Alabama was left to the state to decide. The leaders of Alabama were never to grant that equality. In the same treaty, the U.S. government encouraged the Mvskoke to sell these reserves and move west. The government agreed to pay for the move and for subsistence needs for the first year thereafter. The Mvskoke found that their situation did not improve after the treaty, and violent encounters between the Mvskoke and the Alabamians and Georgians increased. In 1836 a group of angry Mvskoke attacked a group of Alabamians near the Chattahoochee River. President Jackson's reaction was swift. He ordered forced removal west to Indian Territory in 1836 and 1837.[22]

FORCED REMOVAL AND ITS AFTERMATH, 1836–1860
The removal was a bitter experience that the Mvskoke have not forgotten. They have passed down stories of the forced emigration through the generations. Some of these stories were collected in the 1930s as part of the Indian Pioneer Papers Project. Many Mvskoke remembered:

> Many years ago, my grandmother, Sallie Farney, who was among those that made the trip to the West from Alabama, often told of the trip.
> In every way we were abundantly blessed in our every day life in the old country. We had our hunting grounds and all the things that are dear to the heart or interest of an Indian. . . .
> Many of the leaders, when unrest was felt in the homes, visited the different homes and gave encouragement to believe that Alabama was to be the permanent home of the Muskogee tribe.

But many different rumors of a removal to the far West were often heard.

The command for a removal came unexpectedly upon most of us. There was the time that we noticed that several overloaded wagons were passing our home, yet we did not grasp the meaning. However, it was not long until we found out the reason. Wagons stopped at our homes and the men in charge commanded us to gather what few belongings could be crowded into the wagons. We were to be taken away and leave our homes never to return. This was just the beginning of much weeping and heartaches.

We were taken to a crudely built stockade and joined others of our tribe. We were kept penned up until everything was ready before we started on the march. Even here, there was the awful silence that showed the heartaches and sorrow at being taken from the homes and even separation from loved ones.

Most of us had not foreseen such a move in this fashion or at this time. We were not prepared, but times became more horrible after the real journey was begun.

Many fell by the wayside, too faint with hunger or too weak to keep up with the rest. The aged, feeble, and sick were left to perish by the wayside. A crude bed was quickly prepared for these sick and weary people. Only a bowl of water was left within the reach, thus they were left to suffer and die alone.

The little children piteously cried day after day from weariness, hunger, and illness. Many of the men, women and even the children were forced to walk. They were once happy children—left without mother and father—crying could not bring consolation to these children.

The sick and the births required attention, yet there was no time or no one was prepared. Death stalked at all hours, but there was no time for proper burying or ceremonies. My grandfather died on this trip. A hastily cut piece of cottonwood contained his body. The open ends were closed up and this was placed along a creek. This was not the only time this manner of burying was held nor the only way. Some of the dead were placed between two logs and quickly covered by shrubs, some were shoved under the thickets, and some were not even buried but left by the wayside.

There were several men carrying reeds with eagle feathers attached to the end. These men continually circled around the wagon trains or during the night around the camps. These men said the reeds with feathers had been treated by the medicine men.

Their purpose was to encourage the Indians not to be heavy hearted nor to think of the homes that had been left.

Some of the older women sang songs that meant "We are going to our homes and land; there is one who is above and ever watches over us; He will care for us." This song was to encourage the ever downhearted Muskogees.

Many a family was forced to abandon their few possessions and necessities when their horses died or were too weary to pull the heavy wagons any further.

—Mary Hill[23]

* * *

My folks came over with Opuithli Yahola [Opothle Yoholo] from Alabama and stopped at North Fork Town. They left everything they had in the house and walked off. Some sold their possessions. They suffered a lot. I remember the old folks talking at night about the trip, of how they walked until the underneath parts of their feet were bleeding, and they had to limp but kept coming on toward the new land.

—D. W. Benson[24]

* * *

Uncle Willie Benson used to tell me about how they came to this county. When they started out they were afoot and were driven like cattle. At first they had something to eat but that gave out and they were starving. If they had had guns or string they could have gotten game or fish but were not allowed to have them. They came to a slippery elm tree and ate the bark of that until they could get something else. When they would give out they would camp for two or three days to rest up a very little bit, then come on again. Lots took sick and died, so there were not so many when they got here. Big boats were used to haul them across the streams and lakes. When they got to Arkansas they were unable to walk farther so wagons were provided for the rest of the trip. I don't know just where they located first but they were Muskogee Indians under Opothle Yahola.

—Lizzie Wynn[25]

* * *

O-chee Harjo, who was my father, told the story. . . . He said he and his father were along during the sorrowful journey and he

told of the pitiful sights that they saw on their journey. . . . It was
at that time as my father said that my grandfather gave out from
old age and exposure and fell on the way. His grave was a small
brooklet which was chosen because it was rather deep and narrow.
My grandfather's body was placed in this and the dirt picked with
axes from along the banks was then heaped over the body.

—Willie Harjo[26]

The death toll during the removal has been estimated at 3,500. Those
who survived were suffering physically and economically. They were in
such poor physical condition that for the first two years after their arrival
in Indian Territory, scarcely any infants were seen. Women did not con-
ceive and infants died. The estimated Mvskoke population on the eve of
removal was 25,000. Twenty years later in Indian Territory, the Bureau
of Indian Affairs census counted the Mvskoke population at 14,888. The
loss of life in a twenty-year span had been substantial.[27]

The move westward gave the Mvskoke at least temporary rest from
pressure from whites for land. The Treaty of 1832 guaranteed that no
state or territory should ever have a right to pass laws for the government
of the Mvskoke in their new homes. The Mvskoke were promised that
the lands in the West should be theirs "as long as the grass grows and the
rivers run."[28] The Indian Intercourse Act of 1834 forbade unauthorized
entrance into any reservation. This should have safeguarded the Mvskoke
from white encroachment. The impact of whites, however, continued to
be felt in fraud involved in paying annuities and dispersing provisions.
The federal government sent Ethan Allen Hitchcock into the Mvskoke
area in Indian Territory to investigate. He documented numerous cases
of fraud against the Indians, including short weights used for food and
issues of spoiled meat and grain. Hitchcock's report was never released,
and he found himself shunned by the officers of the Indian Service and
by Secretary of War J. C. Spencer.[29]

Many of the Mvskoke focused their anger over the removal on
Christianity and its missionaries. In 1836 Opothle Yoholo asked that
missionaries be expelled from the Mvskoke lands by the U.S. government.
The ruling went into effect. The missionaries, however, were also the
only source of an English education, and some among the Mvskoke had
converted to Christianity and were anxious for their children to receive
such an education. Thus, in 1841 the Mvskoke National Council negotiated a contract with the Presbyterian Church to build a boarding school.
This school, run by Robert Loughridge, opened at Coweta. Loughridge
later published a dictionary of the Creek and English languages.[30]

Other missionary schools followed and in 1848, the council lifted the ban on Christianity.

THE CIVIL WAR, 1860–1866

The Mvskoke rebuilt their lives in the new land, but within twenty-five years, they were again caught in Euro-American politics in a way that would serve to devastate the new world they had built. This time it was the Civil War.

> The Creeks . . . felt that the Indians should really take no part in the war and refused to take action until it was absolutely forced on them. Most of the officials of the tribes leaned toward the Confederacy and it was true that the majority of the Creeks were really in sympathy with the South; however, some felt that if they did not fight with the North, annuities due the Creeks would not be made and for that reason the Creeks were divided.
>
> A treaty was made finally that the Creeks would join the South.
> —Dan Smith[31]

From 1861 to 1866, the tribe had little contact with the U.S. government as their Indian agent, William Garrett, supported the South, and the Union government did not replace him. In 1861 the Confederate leaders met with the Mvskoke to sign a treaty of alliance. While some leaders like Chilly and Daniel McIntosh signed, Opothle Yoholo, leader of the 1837 removal, and others refused. They refused not because they agreed with the Union; in fact, Opothle Yoholo was a slave owner.[32] They refused to sign because they felt the Mvskoke should remain neutral. Agent Garrett, however, organized the Mvskoke into units of the Confederate army. With the Confederates in control of their area in Indian Territory, those opposed to joining the Confederacy were afraid to stay on their lands. In 1861 under the leadership of Opothle Yoholo, several thousand Mvskoke left for Kansas, where the U.S. government had promised them refuge. Reminiscent of the Red Stick War, once again Mvskoke were pitted against Mvskoke. Colonel Cooper, a Texan, led the Indian Confederate troops under Daniel McIntosh in pursuit of Opothle Yoholo and his followers. Three battles took place. Opothle Yoholo's group eventually reached Kansas, starving, freezing, and with livestock and belongings gone. Lindy Scott recalled the stories.

> Tales have been related of how the Indian followers of Opothle Yahola had to suffer much during the intense cold. The leg, arm,

toes or fingers of some of the Indians were lost by being frozen and
they would have to be amputated in the best manner possible. Many
of the Indians walked barefooted in the sleet and snow although
some tried to give protection to their feet by scantily wrapping
them in clothes.

There happened to be one Indian by the name of Dickie among
the group who was generous enough to kill the horse that he rode.
He distributed the meat among his friends or to those who would
take it. Many of them did not refuse.[33]

Ultimately Kansas was harboring six thousand refugees under minimal
conditions. Many died from exposure.[34]

The Mvskoke lands in Indian Territory were a dangerous battle zone.
The families who supported the Confederates also fled to safety by moving
further south. Lizzie Wynn remembered her family's flight.

We got close to Wetumka when he [Daddy] took very sick and
had to be put to bed. We had stopped at an Indian house. The
northern soldiers came to the door and I was standing at the head
of his bed. They told me to move but I thought that if I stayed
there they surely wouldn't shoot him. They shot him and blood and
brains spattered all over me. I wasn't scared but I was mad. After
they had killed him, they left and the old Negro woman said that
they said they would go after some wagons and come back after
us. We covered daddy up and shut the doors and left him laying
in the bed. There was a hill at the back of the house so we ran to
it so that we could get away without being seen. We traveled two
days and nights without food or water and were exhausted when
we came to a little house where an old woman lived. She had some
hominy or rather corn cooked in water. We stayed two months and
were absolutely naked. . . . We started on another and the last part
of our journey [to the Chickasaw Nation]. When we got there some
soldiers from the South gave us some clothes from wagons and fed
us; it almost killed us as we were used to nothing but corn and
water. We stayed where Boggy Depot is for two weeks then they
took us on to the Washita River. . . . My folks stayed in this bottom
land country and helped with the farming and other work there.[35]

The Civil War was devastating to the Mvskoke who had succeeded in
building an economic base in Indian Territory. Much of the war in Indian
Territory was fought on Mvskoke land, resulting in the destruction of

towns and farms and the loss of livestock and crops. After the war the Mvskoke had nothing to salvage but the land itself.[36]

Insisting that all Mvskoke were Confederate allies and enemies, even though as much as half of the population had sided with the North and many Mvskoke had actually fought on the side of the Union, the United States declared the Treaty of 1832 void and forced the Mvskoke to sign a new treaty in 1866. This treaty required them to cede half of their land for settlement by other Indian tribes and by freedmen, the former slaves of tribal members; to allow a railroad to pass through their territory; and to accept a territorial governor under congressional control. In 1867 tribal leaders met again to establish a national government. They adopted a constitution similar to the United States Constitution, although they retained traditional titles for the two houses of their legislative branch of government and, importantly, the political unit remained the traditional Mvskoke *tvlwv* rather than changing to geographic districts.[37] The legislative houses were the House of Kings and the House of Warriors, reflecting the offices in a traditional Mvskoke *tvlwv* ceremonial ground.

FIGHTING FOR THE LAND ONCE AGAIN: THE CIVIL WAR TO ALLOTMENT, 1866–1906

Beginning with the issues surrounding railroad right-of-way secured by the Treaty of 1866 and continuing through the issues of timber sales, cattle grazing, coal mining, and oil drilling rights, the Mvskoke became embroiled in a continuous series of political and economic battles over their vast resources. Their opponents were the U.S. government, corporations, and non-Mvskoke individuals.[38] Pressure on the Mvskoke to allow white expansion into their lands, both in economic enterprises and in land settlement, was intense. They fought white expansion relentlessly. Sukey Charles expressed the frustration: "When white folks would come to the Territory, we would drive them out, but they would come right back again."[39]

Many times the Mvskoke sent representatives to Washington. Many times they employed lawyers to represent their legal rights. In 1870 the first railroad passed through Mvskoke country and soon there were hundreds of Euro-American families within its borders. In 1871 the U.S. Congress passed a bill removing the rights of American Indian tribes to make treaties and attacking their tribal sovereignty. "No Indian nation as a tribe within the territory of the United States shall be acknowledged or recognized as an independent nation, tribe or power with whom the United States may contract by treaty."[40] In 1873 the Mvskoke were forced to cede another parcel of land, this time for a homeland for the Seminole.

At the same time, there was significant internal strife focused principally around the issue of acculturation—the degree to which the people should give up their old ways of government, land tenure, and culture and adopt white ways. In 1889 Pleasant Porter, a Mvskoke leader who was the son of an Irish-American father and a Mvskoke mother from the Perryman family, went to Washington and offered to remove all restrictions on the western lands that had been reserved for Indians and freedmen by the 1866 treaty. This opened the way to white settlement in the western portion of Mvskoke land, and by 1890 it is estimated that of the total Indian Territory population of 210,000 people, 140,000 were white. In 1890 a United States court was established at Muskogee and Congress extended the laws of Arkansas to be applicable in Indian Territory. With this act, the Indians lost the ability to control their lands through the legal system, just as they had sixty years before in Alabama. In 1893, Senator Henry Dawes was appointed by President Cleveland to negotiate with the Mvskoke to extinguish their national title to their land and to arrange for the land to be allotted to individuals. The Mvskoke opposed the proposal. Nevertheless, in 1898 Congress passed the Curtis Act, which terminated tribal jurisdiction, abolished tribal courts, extended jurisdiction of the Dawes Commission over citizenship, made land allotments compulsory, and prohibited payments to tribal governments. Isparhecher, then chief, allowed the question to go to a vote; it was defeated by the Mvskoke people in a general election.[41]

Regardless of this vote, in 1899 the Dawes Commission opened a land office in Muskogee under the authority of the Curtis Act and began the allotment process. Mary Grayson explained, "The Creeks were very much against the Dawes Commission, but couldn't help themselves."[42] Isparhecher was unable to stop the process and lost support. In the same year Pleasant Porter was elected chief. Under Porter, a Mvskoke delegation entered into an agreement with the Dawes Commission. All Indians of Indian Territory became citizens of the United States and the Mvskoke Nation ceased to exist. The U.S. government allowed the office of chief to remain in existence, but the chief became a functionary whose primary role was to sign allotment deeds. The Mvskoke effectively no longer had a government of their own. There were no courts to enforce tribal law and the Indians were under the jurisdiction of the federal government.

Many in the Mvskoke population were angry. A change in the system of land tenure was a primary issue. In 1900 Chief Porter appealed to the federal government for protection against angry Mvskoke, and in 1901 Tcito Hadjo (Crazy Snake), a prominent Mvskoke and former member of the House of Kings, set up a rival government at Hickory Ground *tvlwv*.

His position was that the Treaty of 1832 was still operable and the Mvskoke were governed by it. The "Snakes," the followers of Tcito Hadjo, refused to participate in the allotment process. Forces were sent to quiet them. A confrontation that has become known as the first "snake uprising" ensued.[43] According to Joseph Bruner, in 1901 "a large group of full-blood Creek Indians were dissatisfied with the changes that had been made when the Curtis Act had been passed. As the result of this act the Creek Indians' laws and customs were abolished. The Snake Indians did not want individual allotments but wanted their allotments arranged so the Creek nation could all share equally in the gas, oil and pasture leases."[44]

Regardless, in 1907 the state of Oklahoma, which included Indian Territory, was admitted to the Union. In 1908 all documents, records, and papers of the Mvskoke Nation were turned over to the U.S. Indian Agency at Muskogee, Oklahoma, and the Secretary of the Interior took charge of all tribal property. Dan Smith summed up the Mvskoke loss of resources: "The Creeks after the Civil War received head-right money or bread money. Then they got a few dollars on account of the sale of land to the Arapaho Tribe who were wild Indians and then long before the Dawes Commission was formed they got two payments of maybe $25.00 or maybe $45.00. What the Creeks got other than their allotments of land would not buy a Model T Ford."[45]

In his autobiography, George Washington Grayson provides a glimpse into Mvskoke life during the period from just after removal to statehood. He lived from 1842 to 1920. His father was half Mvskoke and his mother was one-fourth Mvskoke. Grayson was active in Mvskoke politics his entire adult life, eventually serving as chief. In the final paragraph of his autobiography, he wrote of the meaning of the allotment of land and loss of self-government for the Mvskoke.

> Here was a proposal (abolishment of their several tribal governments, the sectionization of their lands, and individualization of the same) that paralyzed the Indians for a time with its bold effrontery. Here we, a people who had been a self-governing people for hundreds and possibly a thousand years, who had a government and administered its affairs ages before such an entity as the United States was ever dreamed of, are asked and admonished that we must give up all ideas of local government, change our system of land holding to that which we confidently believed had pauperized thousands of white people—all for why; not because we had violated any treaties with the United States which guaranteed in solemn terms our undisturbed possession of these; not because of

any respectable number of intelligent Indians were clamoring for a change of conditions, not because any non-enforcement of law prevailed to a greater extent in the Indian territory than elsewhere; but simply because regardless of the plain dictates of justice and a Christian conscience, the ruthless restless white man demanded it. Demanded it because in the general upheaval that would follow the change he, the white man, hoped and expected to obtain for a song, lands from ignorant Indians as others had done in other older states.[46]

STATEHOOD AND LOSS OF TRIBAL SOVEREIGNTY, 1907–1970

After allotment, Indian Territory experienced enormous population growth. The census of 1890 listed 109,393 whites in Indian Territory. The census of 1907 listed 538,512.[47] In less than twenty years, over 400,000 non-Indians had moved onto Indian lands. Land of Indian allottees was restricted from sale, but much of it was leased by whites. After Oklahoma became a state in 1907, the frenzy for Indian resources escalated. In 1908 Congress passed a law that allowed freedmen and mixed-bloods of less than one-half Indian blood to sell their land. Many sold their land willingly. Many others—full-bloods, mixed bloods and freedmen alike—were defrauded. Young allottees were actually kidnapped just before reaching legal age and convinced to sign away their land. Individuals offered to serve as guardians for orphans in order to gain control of their land. In other cases deeds to land were outright forgeries.[48] The discovery of oil increased the pressures. The Glen Pool field and the Cushing field included land of Mvskoke allottees. These rich oil fields led to additional abuses as outsiders and oil companies attempted to gain leases at little cost from Indian individuals. Guardianships of orphans, fraudulent marriages to full-bloods, and various other schemes were used to gain control of Mvskoke wealth. The fight for control of the property of Jackson Barnett is a famous example. Barnett, a former member of the Snake faction, had been allotted land arbitrarily because he refused to participate in the Dawes Commission process. Barnett's allotment turned out to be in the richest section of the Cushing oil field. After his wealth was discovered, he was pursued by prospective marriage partners, and upon his death, there were numerous claims from alleged heirs. His property was tied up in court battles for decades.[49]

In 1932 President Franklin D. Roosevelt had determined that something must be done to arrest the injustices being committed against the Indians. Congress passed the Oklahoma Indian Welfare Act in 1936 in an attempt to stop the fraud. It authorized the tribes to adopt constitutions and to receive charters of incorporation so that they could engage in business, administer tribal property, elect officers, and manage local affairs. A principal chief was appointed by the president but had no power.[50] Several of the traditional Mvskoke *tvlwv* began to explore incorporation for the purpose of acquiring communal land in hopes of returning, to some degree at least, to their traditional form of organization and land tenure.

The 1930s were a difficult time for all people of Oklahoma as the state was hard hit by the Depression. The state's economy was based on agriculture, oil, and coal, and as prices dropped nationally for these products, Oklahomans suffered. One reaction was to overproduce on farmland that was already stressed. The droughts of the early and middle 1930s and the resulting dust storms further crippled the economy and gave Oklahoma the Dust Bowl image familiar to the rest of the country. While the drought was more severe in the northwestern section of the state than in the northeast, where the Mvskoke resided, the entire state experienced severe economic collapse. By the mid-1930s automobile and gas sales began to revive, and by 1937 the rains returned. The 1930s experience, however, gave Oklahomans a near obsessive interest in controlling water, as evidenced in the water control projects of the 1950s and 1960s.[51]

With World War II, life changed for the Mvskoke just as it did for others in the United States. Many Mvskoke joined the U.S. armed forces and afterward many migrated to the cities. Again in the Korean conflict, many Mvskoke served in the armed forces. It was not until 1971 that the Mvskoke finally began to regain control of their own affairs. Estimates are that from the time of statehood in 1907 until 1970, two million acres of land belonging to Mvskoke allottees were sold to outsiders and fifty billion dollars in mineral leases were secured by outsiders. During that period, the Mvskoke had no tribal government to protect their interests.[52]

INDEPENDENCE REGAINED:
THE MUSCOGEE (CREEK) NATION

In 1971 election of the principal chief was returned to the people by congressional authorization. Claude Cox was chosen as chief. The Mvskoke were of differing opinions regarding the way in which representation in a national council should be determined. Many supported representation according to the traditional system of the *tvlwv*. Allen Harjo, who ran against Cox in the 1975 election, was of this opinion. Cox and others supported a new constitution whereby representatives would be elected to one house based on tribal towns and to a second house based on districts. In a 1976 court case, *Harjo v. Kleppe* 420 F. Supp. 1110 (D. D. C. 1976), a U.S. federal district court ruled that the Creek Council established by the 1867 constitution had never been dissolved. In that constitution, tribal towns were the basis for representation. Soon after, in 1979, the Mvskoke adopted a new constitution to replace that of 1867. This constitution was supported by Cox and his followers and had provision for an executive office, a national council of representatives, and a judiciary. While the executive branch of government was in place, the Bureau of Indian Affairs challenged the Nation's right to reestablish its judicial system and refused to fund the tribal courts. In another federal court case, *Muscogee (Creek) Nation v. Hodel*, 851 F. 2d 1439 (D. C. Cir., 1988), the federal district courts gave the Nation the power to establish a judiciary branch, arguing that the Oklahoma Indian Welfare act of 1936 repealed the restrictions on self-government put in place by the Curtis Act of 1898. By 1980, 28,278 people identified themselves as Mvskoke, and 8,766 of them lived in the traditional Mvskoke areas of northeastern Oklahoma.

Now, at the beginning of the twenty-first century, the Muscogee (Creek) Nation is governed by a principal chief, a second chief, a tribal council of twenty-six members elected from eight geographic districts, and a supreme court and district court. The Nation's boundary includes ten counties in Oklahoma. It operates an $82-million-dollar budget and serves 45,860 enrolled tribal members. The Mvskoke are alive and thriving after five centuries of contact.[53]

For centuries the Mvskoke were not a single, unified cultural or political entity but, instead, a group of independent *tvlwv* speaking different languages and with some differences in cultural and religious tradition. The loss of their lands and the attempt to force them to give up their traditional ways brought culture change, including the addition of Christianity. The history of the Mvskoke fight for survival is important to the story David Lewis tells in this book. The centuries of European contact that preceded the forced removal to Indian Territory, the tragedy of that removal, and the century and a half of contact and change that followed are the historical context in which his narrative can be understood.

Chapter Two

HISTORY OF THE LEWIS FAMILY

Lewis's account of his family's history and Jordan's positioning of it in relation to the published and archival material are both presented in this chapter. Lewis's record includes the themes of the forced removal, the ethnic multiplicity of the people now called the Mvskoke, identification with clans, and the importance of medicine in the family's story.

The written tradition provides some information about the three family medicine people who figured most prominently in David Lewis, Jr.'s life: his paternal great grandfather, Jackson Lewis; his father, David Lewis, Sr.; and his maternal grandmother, Jeanetta Jacobs. There are also published references to his own medicine abilities. In the oral tradition that he commits to writing in the chapters to follow, the lives of the members of his family are further defined and interwoven into his own.

DAVID LEWIS, JR.'S PERSONAL NARRATIVE
Father's Family

My great grandfather was Jackson Lewis. He was born in 1837, but that may be wrong. That date is too late. Jackson Lewis made the trip during the removal. He always talked about it. He could remember walking. He was a small child at the time. Alabama is where he came from. And he's not what you would call true Mvskoke either because he said he was a Hitchitee, which is not a Mvskoke.[1] I didn't know him. He's the one who took my dad and taught him everything he knew. Jackson Lewis had eight children and they were good. Daniel, my grandfather, he was a good medicine man; Dad said he was really good, but he was limited. He was never initiated. Jackson Lewis's children were not qualified, so he could never initiate any of his kids even though he shared a lot of things with them up to a certain point. My dad was born and Jackson Lewis took him and taught him everything about the medicine, about how these things originated, and initiated him. Dad said by the time he got to ten he was well on his way—he knew the story of the origin of our medicine in and out.

Dad was small when Jackson Lewis died, anyway. I think Dad said he was ten, almost eleven. And he would talk about how Jackson Lewis was good, how he was powerful. Dad said he saw him do miracles, yet Dad never said what he did. But I saw my dad do things that you could call miracles. So I was always in question, what did Jackson Lewis do? Why was he powerful in the eyes of other people? But you think back, it was a pretty common thing for medicine people because they were all that good. Every one of them, not just one, all of them were good. They were all equal to each other.

Now Jackson, he was a Hitchitee. A lot of the chants I know probably are Hitchitee. Some of them are, I imagine. Because some of the words are not even Creek words. A lot of them are old words anyway. But I couldn't truthfully say that it is Hitchitee because I don't know Hitchitee. So that is what is puzzling, because maybe these are a combination of Hitchitee and Creek words. But then most of the medicine people called our chants "the old words." I don't know which old words they were talking about. We will probably never know. Jackson Lewis always said he was Hitchitee and he was proud of that. He'd say, "I'm not a Creek, I am a Hitchitee." But the record has him down as Creek.

Mother's Family

My grandmother's father was a Seminole. Her dad was a full-blood Seminole. He was a Harjo. He has a roll number on the Seminole roll.[2] But on the record my grandmother is considered a full-blood Mvskoke, which is not true. She was half Mvskoke and half Seminole. The Dawes Commission, the people in charge, put down what they wanted to. I mean the Dawes Commission screwed everything up. I know my grandmother used to laugh, "I was already a teenager when I was born," that is, by her official birth date. How could they miss it by so much? And Indian names, if they couldn't spell them, they just gave them white man's names. That is all they did.

My grandmother never said where her chants came from. She never did talk about it. We did know that she was initiated because she told the story, the same thing that Dad said about how this thing originated. Dad would talk about it; she would talk about it, yet they told the same story, but they were from different grounds. My grandmother was born and raised around Hickory Ground Tribal Town and my dad was from North Canadian Eufaula Tribal Town. They didn't know each other until my dad got married to my grandmother's daughter.

My tribal town is considered to be Hickory Ground and I would be the son of a man from Eufaula. My mother was of the Bird Clan so I am from the Bird Clan. Dad was Turkey Clan. So, it'll still fall under the same as a bird. So, a bird's a bird.

THE FAMILY AND THE WRITTEN RECORD

Turning to the formal historical record, there is substantial information about the medicine people in David Lewis's family. The bringing together of the documents pertaining to the lives of Jackson Lewis, David Lewis, Sr., and Jeanetta Jacobs allows at least parts of those lives to emerge as a written story. Most of the information is of one of the following types: accounts by tribal members; federal government census documents and other rolls enumerating the Mvskoke during the nineteenth- and early twentieth-centuries; and work by anthropologists who interviewed family members.[3]

Paternal Great Grandfather, Jackson Lewis

David Lewis's paternal great great grandparents were Tommie Harjo of Cussetah (Cusseta) Town and Sa Cee Make of Hitchitee Town in the old Mvskoke lands in what is now Alabama and Georgia.[4] Tommie Harjo was killed by a white man in Alabama and buried inside the family home, as was the custom in the old country.[5] John Swanton learned of this in his work with Harjo's son, Jackson Lewis. As Swanton records it:

> Jackson Lewis told me that in Alabama, where he was born, burial inside the house was usual. The grave was dug in one corner flush with the wall, for there were then no floors, and after the body had been placed within, they raised a little house over it, 2 ½ or 3 feet high, and covered it with split planks laid close together. They daubed the sides and top with a thick coating of clay and used the grave as a bed. But before doing so they made some medicine and sprinkled the walls, the ceiling, and in fact the entire house with it in order to counteract any evil influences that might emanate from the body. Jackson Lewis's own father, who had been killed by a white man in the old country, was cared for in this manner.[6]

Tommie Harjo's widow, Sa Cee Make, and son, Jackson, made the journey of the removal from Alabama to Indian Territory. Family members have written about Jackson's experiences during the removal. His shoes wore out from walking and he suffered from cold and hunger. Someone offered him a pony to ride. At the crossing of the Mississippi River, he almost lost his life. The event is related by Chester Scott, his great grandson, and Robert Perry in an account demonstrating that even as a child, Jackson Lewis was already marked by special powers.

> Before his eyes, men and horses were being disastrously carried downstream, pulled under and dragged to the bottom. Jack

nudged his pony into the water, "Let's go." Huge logs were careening down the river. Riders reaching the far bank turned to watch the little boy and his pony. Soon everyone was watching the drama. Midway, something large knocked him from the horse. Jack was swallowing water and gulping for air. No one could help the boy now. Somehow he was able to grab the pony's tail. The horse struggled through the heavy current until he was able to stand and walk to shore. Men lifted the boy in their arms. He had made it! Others who watched the boy's crossing, remarked about seeing a tiny man sitting on the head of that pony. That was strange but the little man was also directing the pony across the raging river with little Jack in tow. . . .

In gratitude, everyone gathered that evening on the west bank. Their tradition was to change the name of a child or man when something important happened in his life. . . . Jack's new name was "Jock-O-Gee" . . . "Gee" means "little." This modest name would mark a small boy who overcame a mighty river. The name had a second unspoken but more powerful meaning. No one had seen the "little people" for at least four generations. Yet, it was clear that the mark of the Great Spirit and the "little people" were on Jock-O-Gee. No one dared to speak the river's name. "Gee" was as close as they dared to speak the full name of the "little people." The Knowledge and protection by the "little people" reside with peace-makers. From the day the river was crossed, "they" were with Jock-O-Gee, teaching him how to doctor sick people in the new land with new herbs and plants.[7]

Hence Jackson Lewis's reputation for a powerful connection with the spirit world begins with stories from his childhood; the little people mentioned in this narrative are revered spiritual entities among traditional Mvskoke.

The terrible experiences of the removal are remembered by the Lewis family, as David Lewis, Jr., recounts:

I believe that this part of the story I will tell is very important because it brings out the true feelings of my great grandfather, Jackson Lewis. It shows how he felt about his old home place after he had established his home in this new country, Oklahoma. Jackson Lewis more than once said to my dad that he really didn't have any feeling for the old home place; to him it didn't exist in his heart. He told Dad that when the time of leaving was upon his family, most of the things that belonged to them that couldn't be carried, his dad (Harjo) told his family to bury them three feet down or more.

As they were getting ready to leave, his dad (Harjo) gathered the family and put his arms around them. He talked to the family and instructed them, "Don't look back. Don't look back. The beauty you once saw is no longer there. The beautiful sound of singing from the birds you once heard is silence forever. The soft music the leaves of the trees made as the wind blew gently will never fall upon your ears again. All of these things that you once loved and knew are gone forever. They no longer exist today. What we have here today is something that we should all remember and always carry in our hearts. Pass this heartache and sorrow that this family experienced down to your children." My dad, David Lewis, Sr., said he could remember the sad look in Jackson Lewis's eyes as Jackson Lewis put his arms around Dad after telling that story and said, "These are the things that happened in our family's life; you must remember this story and carry this in your mind and heart just as I have and pass this down to your children and their children."

It is well known in the Lewis family that our great grandfather, Jackson Lewis, had no tie or feeling for the old home place in Alabama, but he did want to go back to the great river where he almost drowned while crossing to come to this new place, called Oklahoma.

By his own account, Jackson Lewis and his mother did not reach the Mvskoke area in Indian Territory until 1847. While most of the Mvskoke left the Southeast in large groups with government escort in the years 1836, 1837, and 1838, individuals and small groups continued to remove at their own expense until 1842. The Treaty of 1832 promised that all individuals would be recompensed for the expense of removal and given money for subsistence for one year after arrival. An attempt was made to identify those who removed at their own expense in order that they might be reimbursed by the government. The roll developed for this purpose by Judge G. W. Stidham in 1886 includes the names of Jackson Lewis, age six, and his mother, Sa Cee Make, from Hitchitee town. Attached to it is the following sworn statement taken from Jackson Lewis in 1886 and recorded as proof of the move:

I live in the Indian Territory, and am enrolled in Hitche-tee town, on the list of G. W. Stidham. . . . [M]y name is entered or enrolled as Jackson (m), six year old, which is a mistake. I am about fifty-five years of age. The statement as to our emigration is correct in part, but it fails to show that the family stopped for several years in the Choctaw Nation, near Doaksville. We paid our own expenses, and are entitled to transportation and subsistence for twelve months after our arrival.[8]

Thus, it is not possible to determine when or under what circumstances the family left the Southeast. What is known from the above document is that the family stayed for an undetermined amount of time in the Choctaw Nation and arrived in the Mvskoke area in 1847. Jackson Lewis's aside about his age being fifty-five years is a reference to the time of the sworn statement, not the removal.

He grew to adulthood in Indian Territory and was by all accounts a well respected individual—a ball player, a hunter, and a business entrepreneur. His grandson, David Lewis, Sr., remembered:

> His first venture was the establishment of a store that was called Tulofa Chule (Old Town). It was located right east of the present site of Eufaula and before Eufaula was ever begun. There was everything to sell at that store, mostly the things that were in demand and in use of those days. Many whites and Indians came to trade at Tulofa Chule by way of oxen or horse team and wagons, horseback and walking. He had quite a bit of active business there because Jackson Lewis was a genial and friendly man to everyone. He was wont to extend too much credit to the Indians and his friends so that this custom eventually led to his downfall in the business causing his bankruptcy.[9]

He then set up a blacksmith shop, making all the tools for it himself. He made axes, chisels, picks, and shovels, even a complete wagon. He also made jewelry out of copper pennies and celluloid combs. Above all, however, he was respected for his medicine abilities. According to David Lewis, Sr., "He had become a medicine man, with calls quite frequent among the Indians for he was noted for his doctoring and his ability to cure serious burns and poisonous insect bites."[10]

Only eighteen years after reaching the Mvskoke area in Indian Territory and at the approximate age of twenty-three, Jackson Lewis, like all the Mvskoke, was caught up in the events of the Civil War. His grandson recalls that "it was at risk of life if any man or Indian youth was found at home so they felt safer doing service as a soldier."[11] Jackson Lewis joined the Confederacy, serving in Company K, second regiment, of the Creek Volunteers.[12] He entered the service in September of 1861 as a first sergeant and by the end of the war had achieved the rank of second lieutenant. As a respected medicine person, he served in the Confederacy in the capacity of an Indian doctor. His great grandson Chester Scott wrote: "He was a good doctor. When an Indian would get shot in the arm by noon-time, the doctor had him ready for battle the next day."[13] He was present at the Battle of Honey Springs in 1863.[14] He told his family stories of his war experiences. David Lewis, Sr., related:

> I have never heard of an Indian having operated a steamboat on a river, although they have built and been in charge of bridges and ferries, but my grandfather of Eufaula town, Jackson Lewis, used to tell of having operated a steamboat on the Arkansas River to haul supplies from Fort Smith to Fort Gibson while in the service for the Confederates. He would tell of how his boat received hails of bullets from either side of the river from the guns of the scattered men of the Union. He said they would sometimes go through with their boat or they would sometimes return to Fort Smith, where more men would board for protection to the boat.[15]

In another story, Jackson Lewis and another Mvskoke soldier were riding double on the same horse trying to reach Eufaula to call for reinforcements. They were pursued and shot from the rear. Later they discovered a bullet that had entered the rear part of the saddle and lodged in the saddle horn without touching either man.[16]

Jackson Lewis survived the war and eventually returned to the Eufaula area, where he belonged to Canadian Eufaula Tribal Town. As was the traditional custom with the Mvskoke, he had several names conferred upon him as a result of deeds done. Other than the name of Jock-O-Gee or Cakocee (Little Jack) that he acquired after crossing the Mississippi River as a child, he also had the name Lahta Yahola, a Creek war name. In addition, he received titles or names that entitled him to certain seats in the Eufaula Square Ground. John Swanton records some of these: "When my informant Jackson Lewis grew to manhood he received the name Tcowasta'I tstngi [*tvstvnvke*], which entitled him to a seat in the south or Warriors' bed at Eufaula, a seat different from the one he had up to that time occupied. In 1908 he received a third name, Ah'lk tstngi, but he kept the same seat."[17]

In the Dunn roll of 1867 for Canadian Ufaula Tribal Town and the 1890 and 1895 census rolls for Eufaula Canadian Town, Jackson Lewis appears as Larter Yarholar or Lahta Yaholer—altered spellings of Lahta

Yahola, just as Eufaula and Ufaula were altered spellings for the name of the same tribal ground. Frequently, Indian names were spelled in a variety of ways in official documents. An official alphabet of the Creek language had been adopted in 1853, but most whites and many Indians who had occasion to write the language were unfamiliar with the official spellings and simply wrote the words as they saw fit.[18] The difficulty whites had with Indian names, and their need to establish exact identities and family relations of all Mvskoke in order to issue allotments, led to the use of the English patrilineal naming system to identify Mvskoke individuals. Thus Indian names were changed to English names with families identified by a patrilineal family name. The Mvskoke lost, for legal purposes, their traditional names and naming system and their matrilineal kinship reckoning to the English system more easily understood by the whites. The English name Jackson Lewis first appears in the written record on the roll created by Judge Stidham in 1886 and appears again later on Lewis's allotment documents of 1901 and 1902.[19] Lewis married Hannah Proctor and they had seven children, one of whom was Daniel, the grandfather of David Lewis, Jr. Later Jackson Lewis married Nancy Walton and they had one daughter.[20]

Jackson Lewis lived a long and honorable life. He was baptized in 1856 and in 1861 he joined West Eufaula Church, an Indian Baptist Church, where he long served as a deacon. He was made a Mason in 1863 and continued to be active in the Masons for most of his life. He was a trustee of West Eufaula School in 1884. He served in the Creek National Council, representing Eufaula Canadian Town in the House of Warriors in 1886, 1892, and 1897. He served in the House of Kings in 1893.[21] Throughout his life he was renowned as a traditional medicine doctor. His visit to Muskogee in 1908 occasioned an article in the local newspaper. Under the headline, "Some Pumpkins on Writing Creek," the *Times-Democrat* declared: "Although unable to speak or write a word in English, Jackson Lewis, an aged full blood Creek Indian, who is visiting in Muskogee, enjoys the distinction of being the only one among 11,000 members of his tribe who can write the Creek language correctly. Lewis lives near Eufaula."[22]

Shortly before his death, Lewis was interviewed extensively by John Swanton, ethnographer with the Bureau of American Ethnology. Swanton identifies him as a leading informant and refers repeatedly to his fine reputation as a person and as a doctor with descriptions like "Jackson Lewis, a Hitchiti doctor who stood high in the estimation of both Indians and whites" or "Jackson Lewis whose evidence is always valuable" or "Jackson Lewis, one of my oldest and best informants."[23] As already noted, the importance of Lewis's contributions to Swanton's classic work *Religious Beliefs and Medical Practices of the Creek Indians* is evidenced by the numerous references Swanton makes to Lewis and to the value of his information.[24]

Lewis died in 1910. At his death, George W. Grayson, who had known him since boyhood, served with him in the Civil War, and was present at some of the interviews with Swanton, wrote of Lewis: "He was a good man. Gentle as a lamb, always considerate and contributive to the comfort of those about him, he was the embodiment of the true Christian gentleman. . . . Thus disappeared from the stage of action one who in a sense was a truly great man. I only wish that at my death there could be someone who could say as many favorable things of one conscientiously, as I can of Jackson Lewis."[25]

Jackson Lewis's grandson, David Lewis, Sr., wrote in his personal family records:

Jackson Lewis Enrollment Name C. 7131
Cakoccee Harjo. Before Enrollment Name.
Born—About 1837 in the State of Alabama.
Died. December 21—1910. Age 73 years.
Member, West Eufaula Ind. Church.
Baptized—March 23, 1856.
Deacon—Ordained—1861.
He was Indian Doctor.
He was fought—1860–65—Civil War.
He was a—"Democrat."
Have Eight Children.

In an interview with a local newspaper, David Lewis, Sr., said: "My grandfather, Jackson Lewis, was able to predict storms and cure all kinds of ailments. . . . I learned a lot from him. I listened well to his words. He told me not to smoke or drink. It would hurt my brain and I could not understand the little folk and be able to cure sickness."[26]

Father, David Lewis, Sr.

Jackson Lewis's son Daniel (1867–1922) married Polly Thompson (1870–1965) in Indian Territory in 1883. They had nine children, four of whom died in childhood. David B. Lewis, Sr. (1899–1985), was the fifth child. He grew up in the Artussu Indian community southwest of Eufaula, Oklahoma, and attended a one-room school near there. The school closed soon after the beginning of World War I, when Lewis had finished the

fifth grade. He later married Sallie Jacob of Hickory Ground and moved
to her home area outside Henryetta. They raised two daughters and one
son, David Lewis, Jr. Sallie Jacob Lewis died in 1935 when her son was a
small child. David Lewis, Sr., returned to his community of Artussu and
spent the last years of his life living in one of the camp houses at the West
Eufaula Indian Church with his brother, Washi. Traditional Mvskoke-
style Indian church grounds contained a church building surrounded by a
number of camp houses in which the members cooked and resided during
church meetings.[27]

Like his grandfather, David Lewis, Sr., was well recognized for his ability
as a medicine man. He was the subject of an article in the local newspaper in
Muskogee, Oklahoma. In the article he talked about medicine:

> Indian medicine is stronger than white man's medicine because
> the little people know exactly what the sickness is. . . . The little
> people first came to me when I was being initiated as a boy. Since
> then they have been with me. They live in the pine tree outside my
> home. I planted that pine tree myself many long years ago. In the
> early mornings, they crawl down from their hiding places among
> the tree bark and come to my shoulder to speak to me. They tell me
> of people who are coming to see me and sometimes how I should
> treat their sickness. . . . Indian medicine is very strong. The little
> folk tell me what the sickness is and the potions for the cure. I then
> go to the woods hoping to find the proper herb, flower or seed to
> mix. Sometimes I cannot find them and I have to look in the woods
> far away from here. The little folk can tell about tornadoes, too.
> Somewhere the evil spirits have torn the tail from the old water
> turtle and it is spinning causing the winds to turn. There are mix-
> tures to be sprinkled in the house to keep the winds away. . . . If
> you live long enough, you can get the answers to everything you
> question. . . . I'm getting too old to get to the woods to gather the
> herbs for people. The doctor woman says I should not go into the
> woods. I might drop dead and no one would know where I am. I
> think that's what happens to the little folk—they get old and they
> wander off from the pine trees into the woods, to the West.

Of his own son, David Lewis, Jr., he said, "He will make a pretty good
medicine man."[28]

Maternal Grandmother, Jeanetta Jacobs
David Lewis, Jr.'s matrilineal family is also documented in written records,

although less thoroughly. In the matrilineal clan of which he is a member, his maternal great grandparents were Semi-hoye of the Bird Clan and Hickory Ground Tribal Town and Arbarthlee Harjo of the Raccoon Clan. Semi-hoye died before the Civil War. She had six children, three daughters with an earlier husband and two daughters and a son with Arbarthlee Harjo. One of the daughters born to Semi-hoye and Arbarthlee Harjo was Jeanetta, David Lewis, Jr.'s grandmother.

Confusion exists in the government enrollment records. Arbarthlee Harjo married Semi-hoye and two of her daughters by a previous marriage. This marriage pattern, in which a mother and her daughters might be married to one man, was traditionally common among the matrilineal Mvskoke. It resulted, however, in great confusion at the time the Dawes land allotment census was taken. In the allotment census, Euro-American census takers recorded Mvskoke people as if they reckoned descent patrilineally. The fact that Arbarthlee Harjo, renamed Arbuckle, had as his three wives a mother and her two daughters from a previous marriage and that a matrilineally related family unit living together also included Arbarthlee Harjo's grandchildren was too confusing for the white census takers to understand. It resulted in two of his grandchildren receiving two allotments of land each, as they were recorded inaccurately as Harjo's children and also accurately as the children of their actual father, who did not reside in the same family unit.[29]

Jeanetta married Sam or Shawnee Jacobs. His mother was of the Tiger Clan and was from Hickory Ground and his father was of the Fox Clan and from Tuckabatchee. Sam Jacobs was, therefore, of Hickory Ground. Jeanetta and Sam Jacobs's daughter, Sallie, married David Lewis, Sr. Sallie and David Lewis, Sr., had three children, two daughters and a son. The son was David Lewis, Jr.

Jeanetta Jacobs enjoyed a reputation as a powerful medicine woman. In interviews collected with Mvskoke during the 1930s as part of the Indian Pioneer Papers Project, two individuals interviewed mention her as a medicine person. Linda Collins of Thlocco Town explained that "the Indian women used medicine at the grounds every year and so were healthy. Most of them didn't need doctors but if they had a hard time there were women doctors who assisted them. There are women doctors still living, Jenetta Jacobs lives close to the Hickory Ground Church." Mary Freeman of Eufaula-Hitchita Town stated, "Jenata Willie, Jenata Jacobs and Annie Lechlie were Indian doctors that I knew of."[30]

The anthropologist Alexander Spoehr interviewed Jeanetta Jacobs in his study of Mvskoke kinship conducted in 1938 and 1939. At the time, David Lewis, Jr., would have been a small boy living in the same home.

Spoehr's field notes with Jeanetta Jacobs state: "Mrs. Jacobs is an elderly
woman who knows the kinship system backwards and forwards. She married an Osochi [Hickory] man, who is now dead. She also has a reputation
as being a very good doctor." Spoehr used information he learned from
Jeanetta Jacobs in his work on Mvskoke kinship.[31]

David Lewis, Jr.

References to the medicine work of David Lewis, Jr., are also found in
the written record. He was born in 1933, into the matrilocal household
described above. The family lived in a house belonging to his grandmother
built on land in McIntosh County that had been allotted to her under the
Curtis Act. After his mother's death, David Lewis, Jr., continued to live
with his sisters in his grandmother's home until he was about eleven when
he was enrolled in an Indian orphanage home in Muskogee, Oklahoma.
Throughout his early childhood, his grandmother and father both worked
extensively with him, training him in the medicine tradition.

As a young man, he left northeastern Oklahoma. He attended Haskell
Institute (now Indian Nations University) in Lawrence, Kansas. In 1954,
he joined the U.S. Marine Corps and served in the Korean conflict. He
returned to civilian life in 1959 with an honorable discharge and soon
afterward attended the Northrup Institute of Technology in Inglewood,
California, to study aircraft repair. He then returned to the Southwest and
was employed as a shop foreman working on Bell helicopters in Fort Worth
and Arlington, Texas. Lewis states, "No matter where I went, I always knew
I would come home, that my place was here." He did indeed return home
to Oklahoma, where he joined his father as a medicine man and worked
in various tribal endeavors for both the Muscogee (Creek) Nation and
the Chickasaw Nation. He returned to school and received an Associate
of Science degree at Connors State College in Warner, Oklahoma in 1979
and a Bachelor of Arts from East Central University in Ada, Oklahoma in
1981. In 1994 he was elected to the Muscogee (Creek) Nation National
Council, where at the time of this writing he is serving his fifth term. He
is married and has four children and five grandchildren.

Since the age of nine, when he made medicine for a client for the first
time, his primary occupation has been serving as a medicine man. He
travels throughout the United States in this capacity and also lectures on
the subject of traditional medicine culture. In 1993 he was interviewed
by Maura McDermott for an article on American Indian medicine for
Oklahoma Today, the official magazine of the state of Oklahoma. In that
interview Lewis explained, "A lot of the fancy medicines we buy at the
store for a fancy price contain the same ingredients the Indians used in

the pre-scientific days." He further made it clear that his medicine combined "the use of our sacred words and the plants." McDermott wrote: "Possibly, the cures for some of our most intractable diseases—cancer, Alzheimer's, AIDS—will be found in plants long used by Native Americans. If this should happen, it won't surprise David Lewis, as his faith in the healing power of plants is complete. Long ago, he said, the plants struck a bargain with his people: 'You do your half,' promised the plants, 'and we'll do our half.'"[32]

David Lewis, Jr.'s reputation as a medicine person is also reflected in the *Muscogee Nation News*, the official publication of the Muscogee (Creek) Nation, in several letters to the editor. In the following example, Deanne Bar of Reserve, Kansas, wrote of the help Lewis gave her daughter.

> We have traveled a long, hard road to find a miracle for our daughter Tiffany. . . . We found nothing but heartache and no results. The doctors never could tell us what was wrong with our daughter. Finally they put her on a vegetables-only diet. She had dark circles under her eyes and would not gain weight. Some days she would not have the energy to even walk, so we would have to carry her. As a last resort, the doctors placed her in a behavioral hospital.
>
> That's when we decided we had to look for something that would not hurt her and have lasting effects on her health. We contacted a fellow tribal member who gave us the contact for the miracle. You have the miracle in your medicine man Dave Lewis. We have our daughter back after everyone else had given up hope.
>
> She is gaining weight and has the energy that we thought we would never see again. One thing Lewis could give us, that no medical doctor could, was the caring and goodness of his heart.[33]

In another letter to the *Muscogee Nation News*, Mrs. H. Craig Platt of Dewey described a rash her husband had on his face, neck, chest, and back for four months. After trying medical doctors, they went to David Lewis.

> David came to see my husband and gave him medicine to drink. Within four days, the scales, pus, and scabs had begun to slough off. Even though he still has some small amount of rash left on his neck, face, and scalp, the horrendous sores are gone. His chest and back are clear.
>
> From the earth our Creator gave us natural things to assist us in healing and through medicine men such as David Lewis it is possible.[34]

McDermott, the author of the article in *Oklahoma Today*, described Lewis as "a congenial man with short gray hair and steel-rimmed glasses. . . . Like a small-town doctor, he takes calls from people—Indian and non-Indian alike—who need his services; many are people who are desperate and have tried everything else."[35]

THE LIVING MEDICINE

TRADITION

David Lewis, Jr.

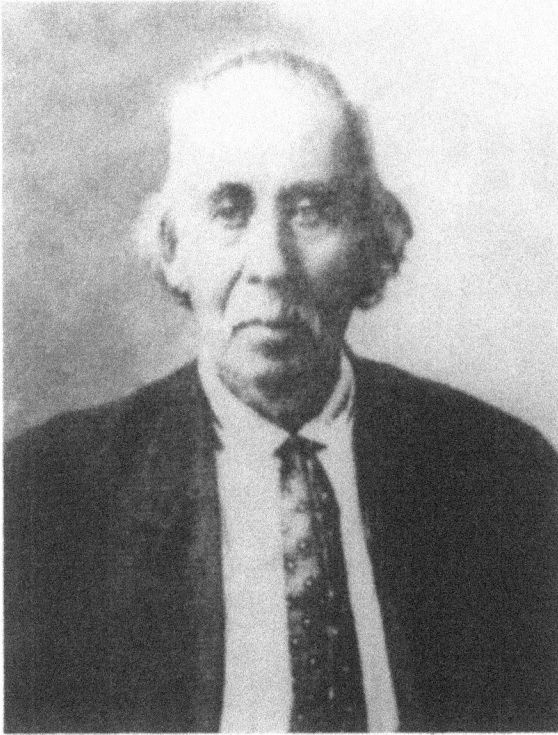

Jackson Lewis, my great grandfather.

Jeanetta Jacobs, my grandmother, is second from the left.

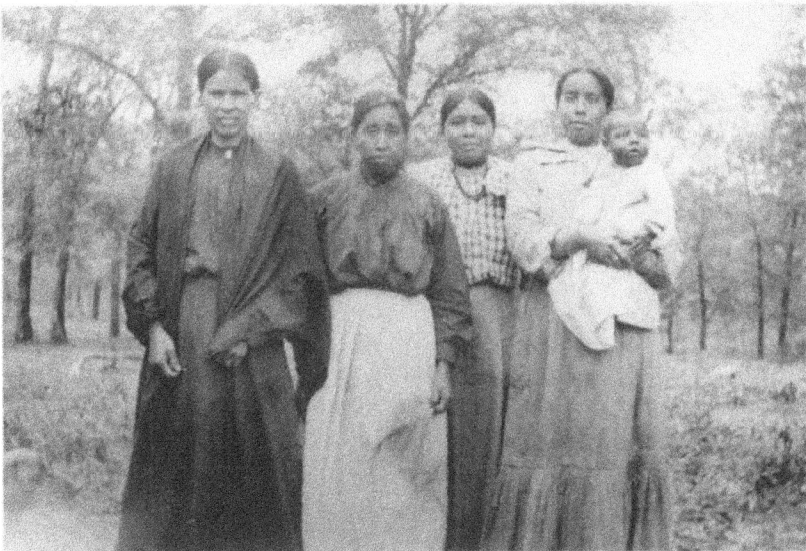

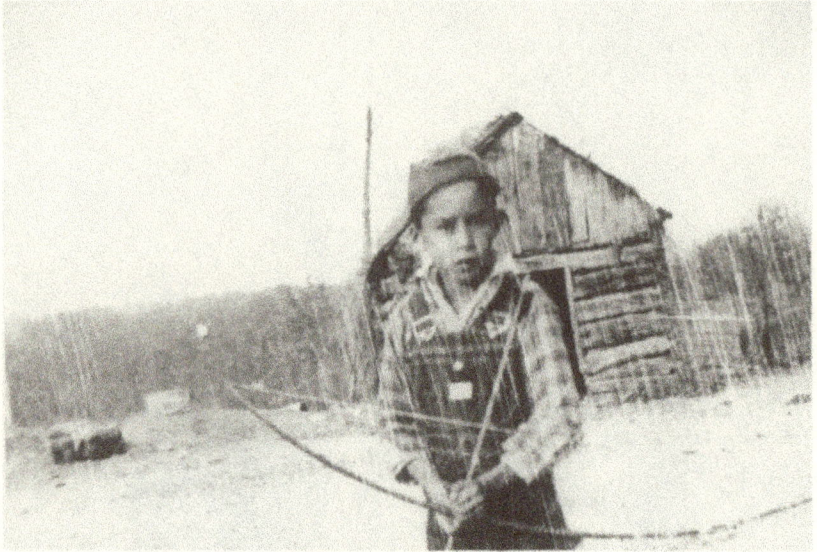

Here, I was about six. This was at my grandmother's, in front of the smoke house.

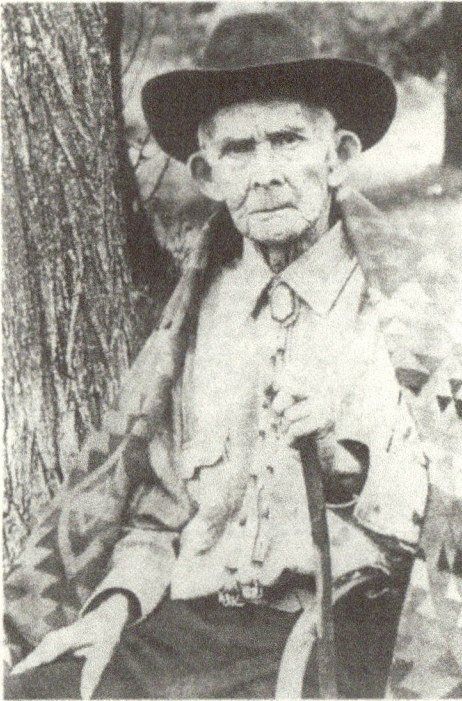

David Lewis, my father.

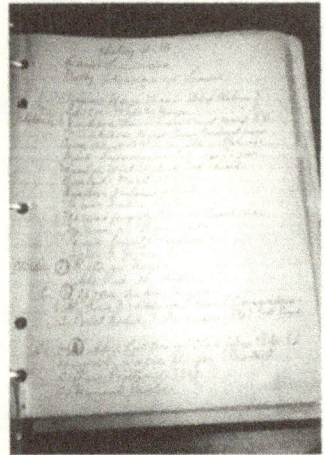

My dad's family tree. He wrote this down many years ago.

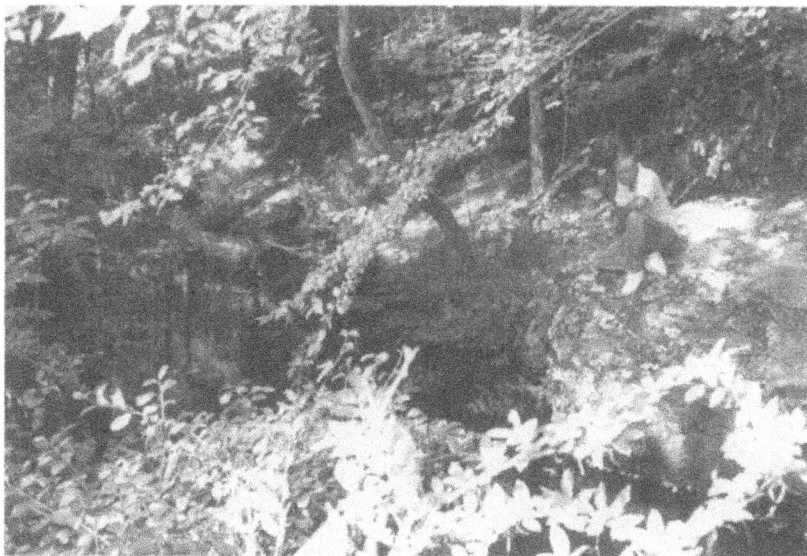

Initiation. I am looking down into the water where my grandmother initiated me.

Initiation. I am sitting right by the mystery rock. I have my hand on that rock.

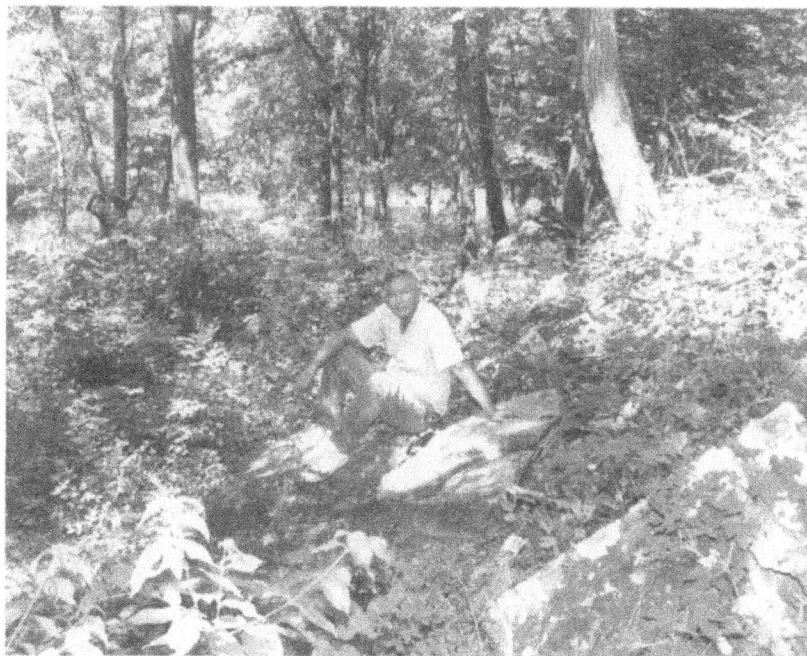

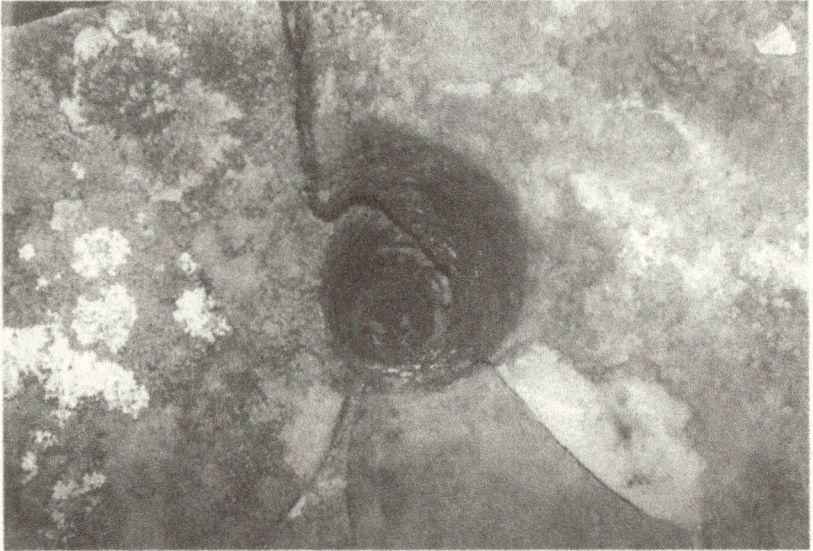

Initiation. The mystery rock, shoved back together. It shows that little cylinder that the medicine was in.

Initiation. My dad initiated me here. I am standing where I was standing when he shoved me into the water.

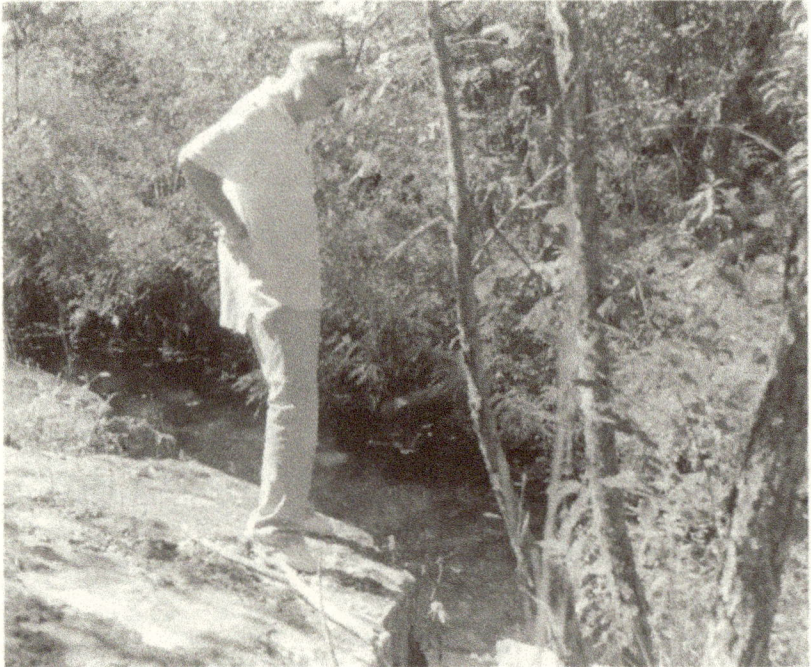

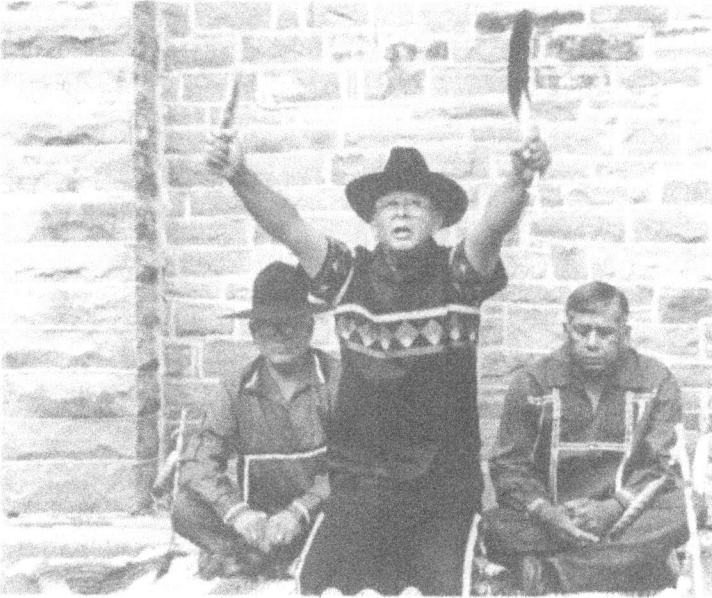

Blessing Ceremony. I am giving thanks to the Creator and opening heaven's door for the deceased to join us on that special occasion. You can see the four poles outlining the sacred square.

Blessing Ceremony. This is the blessing, starting on the north side of the old Creek Council House. My two assistants are with me.

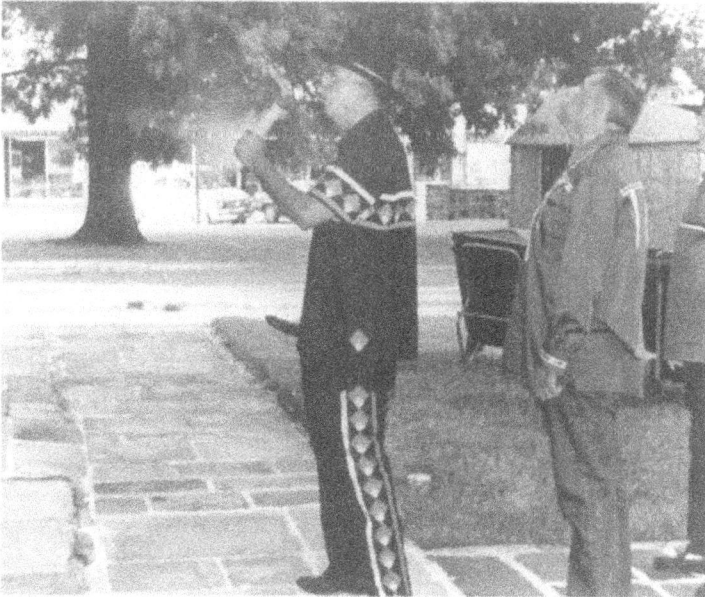

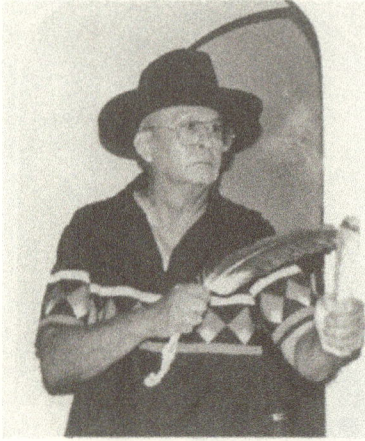

Blessing Ceremony.
I am smoking out the inside
of the council house, blessing it.

This is the little horn.
It is about four inches long.

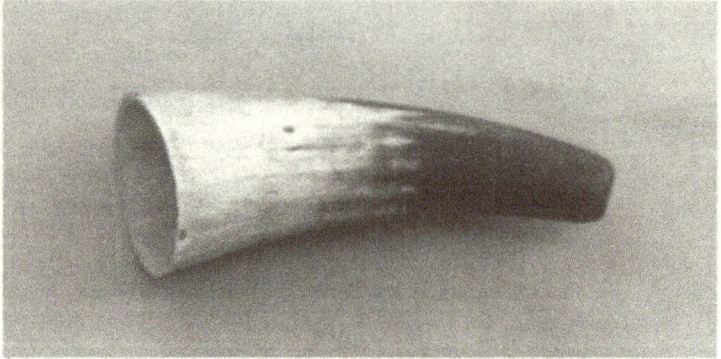

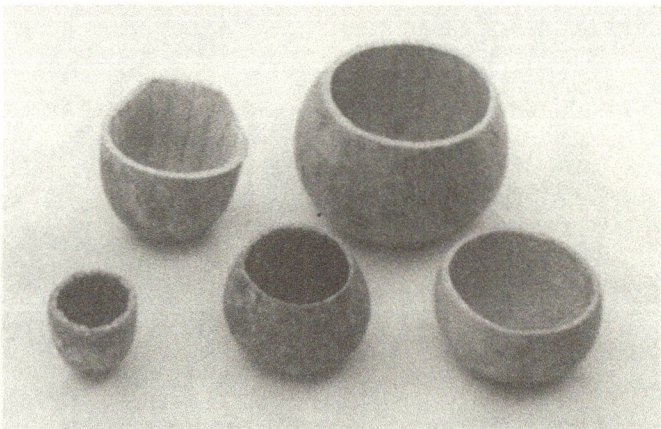

These are measuring cups. The biggest one is probably about four
inches in diameter and the smallest is an inch. They are very small.
The one on the top left is for a baby.

My sacred poles to mark the sacred square. They are three to four feet long. You don't want them to be obvious, so you want them short. That way someone walking by won't see them.

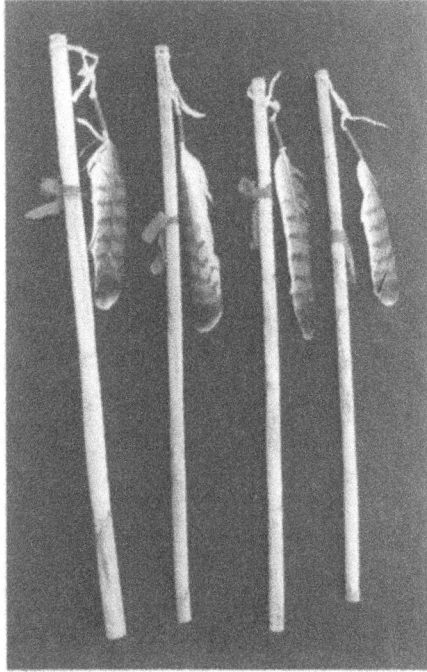

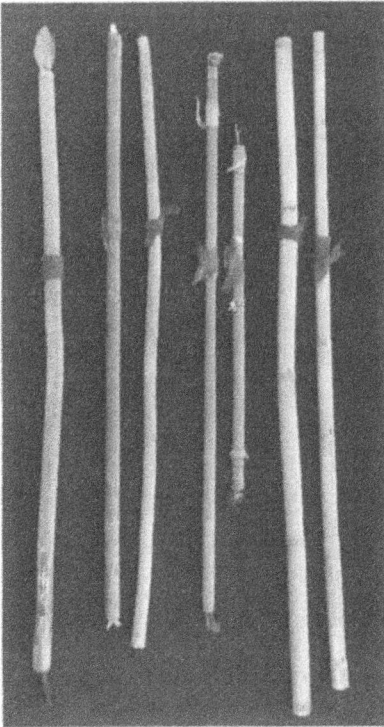

These are medicine sticks. They are usually about thirty inches long. The shortest one in this picture is probably about eighteen inches long. From left to right they are:

— The one my great grandfather, Jackson Lewis, gave to my dad.
— The one Dad gave to me after I was initiated.
— The one Dad used the most after giving the other one to me. He used it until he died.
— The one my grandmother gave to me after I was initiated.
— The one she used until the day she died.
— The one I use the most when I'm using my dad's words.
— The one I use the most when I'm using my grandmother's words.

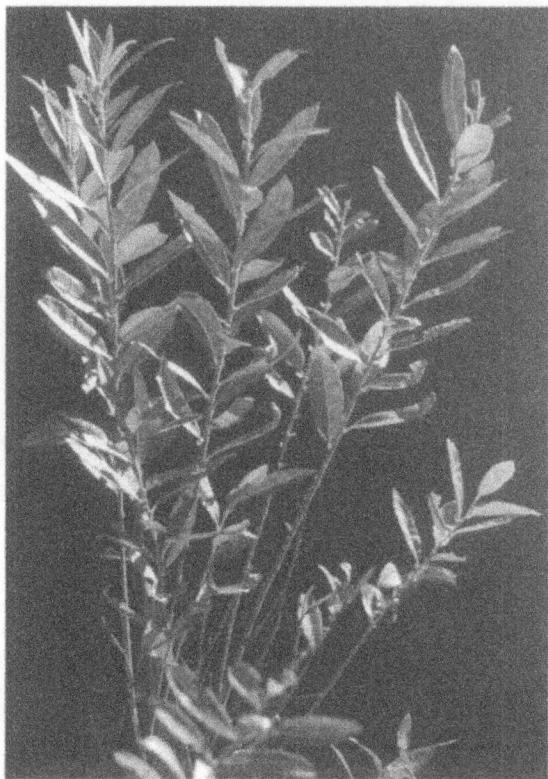

*Red root plant,
mᵛekko-hoyvnecv.*

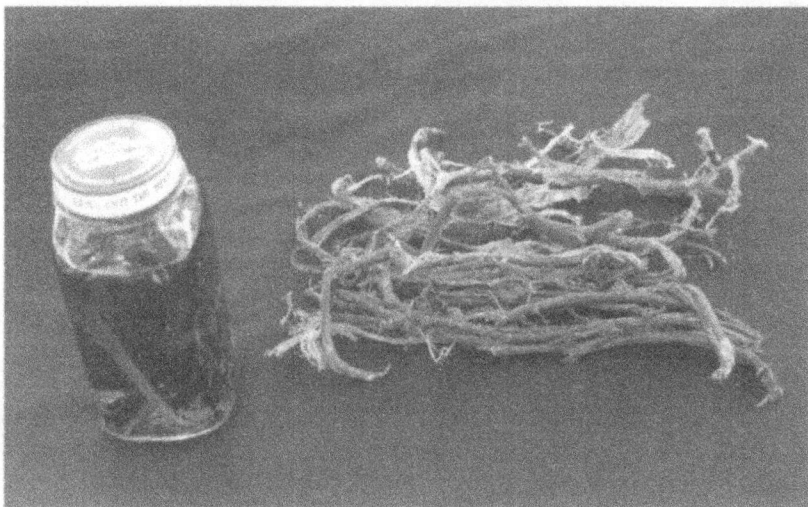

*Red root. The bark has been stripped from the roots and is ready to use.
The jar shows what it looks like when you put the roots in water.*

Chapter Three

KINDS OF MEDICINE PEOPLE

The use of medicine was a dominant force in the lifestyle and in the ceremonial rituals of the ancient Mvskoke people. It is said that knowledge and the use of songs and herbs, to some limited extent, was practiced by the majority of the old Mvskokvlke long ago. There was medicine for nearly everything that affected Indian people, such as health, physical strength, mental well-being, peace, social well-being, family and home well-being, war, and even important speaking. All things that influence life and death were dealt with sacredly and religiously through the God-given powers of the medicine ways. Among the Mvskoke people, the *heles-hayv* (medicine maker) is the medicine person and there are three types.

THE MAIN Heles-Hayv

This medicine person, who could be a man or woman, was the highest in status among the medicine people and commanded the greatest respect. This person was chosen from an early age. As the chosen child developed, he or she was watched, tutored, and, if need be, disciplined. Contrary to modern belief, the Mvskoke medicine people did not have medicine schools for group instruction. Some of the qualities looked for in the child were good temperament, being prone to fairness and good judgment, seriousness, and an exceptional ability to understand.

The child in this category was generally gifted and possessed certain mystic or psychic abilities, which allowed diagnostic insights. If the child was gifted, then he or she could be an *owalv* (prophet or seer) or a *kĕrrv* (one who knows). This child could either be born with this gift or develop it as the child grew under the supervision of the main *heles-hayv* who was to train the child as his or her sole replacement. This status of a main medicine person was usually inherited through the family. Yet there were provisions when there was no family to continue the status.

A main *heles-hayv* was generally consulted by the lesser classes of medicine people. They were, for the most part, not active in social or ceremonial ritual affairs of the Mvskoke people, but maintained a rigorous, disciplined lifestyle in order that the powers of their gifts would be effective for the people they served.

One of the main qualifications in this class was that of special initiation.

After having completed the instruction and rigors of preparations, the candidate would then go through the special initiation that authorized his or her place as a medicine person in this class. Now the potential was confirmed into mystic ability and he or she would be responsible to the calling that would be fulfilled sometime in his or her life.

The main medicine person instructed the chosen child. Every time the candidate learned something good to cure, then they learned the other one, the opposite, destructive. So every time you learn a cure, they'll teach you another one that'll be just the opposite, that you can totally ruin everything if you want to. That's why with the chosen child they had to know whether he or she would misuse the medicine, use it the wrong way, hurt people. They can't give the one being trained as the sole replacement of a main *heles-hayv* just all good.

Once the main medicine people are gone we'll never keep up with the times like it has been in the past, all these hundreds of years. There'll be new things coming in, like the AIDS, that there'll be no cure for from an Indian point of view, anymore. There'll be no visions. No plants to be shown. Only the main *heles-hayv* has the visions that show new cures.

THE CARRIER

The medicine person in this category is also called *heles-hayv*, but is one who has acquired medicine knowledge through their own interest and may be a learner or a disciple of a main *heles-hayv*. Their knowledge may also be developed by seeking knowledge from other medicine people. A carrier may possess the unique mystic qualities that are generally associated with the main *heles-hayv*. Carriers may or may not be associated with the ceremonial grounds or with a Christian church. There is no initiation in this category, but in all cases, in order to affect the positive well-being of the people they serve, they must seek to live as pure as possible. This is the ideal standard for all medicine people.

The carriers could learn nothing but good. For a carrier you select a person who's going to carry on from your side of the family. It doesn't have to be a relative; you've just got to know that the person will carry out your instructions about how it's supposed to be done. And then, you could also initiate that person or persons up to a certain point where you'll teach them certain things. And you can teach them nothing but good, but remember they're limited. What you'll give them is all they'll ever know. They'll never see any visions to learn new medicines. So, they're limited. Carriers do have an advantage because you teach them to do nothing but good, unlike the main medicine people.

For instance, Jackson Lewis's children were carriers so they were limited. They were just as strong as he was because of one thing. Everything that the main *heles-hayv* would teach about one cure, the carrier would be just as strong as the medicine person who taught him or her in that one cure. You give them everything you've got. You are giving them permission to carry the words of your family. That is why he or she is called a carrier, because they carry the words of a main *heles-hayv*. There are procedures that you put all your carriers through. A medicine man who is going to share something with another person, who is going to make a person a carrier, he would make medicine for that person to use for at least four days. The medicine man and the person who is going to learn would already have a day set to meet that they will get real serious about the training. The medicine man has this person purified, cleaned off, and then he uses another medicine on the person so that the person will be ready to receive words. The medicine man that is going to teach also has himself prepared. He is prepared to give the sacred words out. Both persons must use medicine. That is why I won't talk about the medicine with anybody because I don't do that if I am not prepared. And a carrier could share the sacred words with another carrier if the carrier has been properly prepared.

What I see now is that our medicine is getting weaker because the people that have shared things with other people, they were not prepared. It just doesn't happen anymore, maybe because of the hard work involved in getting prepared or because a weak medicine man is trying to teach. In the old way none of the words were written or recorded and now they are and that is not right. In the right way, a person does not have to write it or record it because the person is prepared and when they receive the words, they will know them and not forget. I will hardly read a book that somebody wrote about Indians. I never read another medicine man's words. They say, "Dave you want to read it?" I say, "I don't read other people's books, what somebody else has." I just tell them in a nice way that I don't want to see that. I don't even let them talk about it. You never talk about medicine unless you are prepared anyway and there is nothing they can give me. I'm not interested. But I am always nice though.

If you bother a medicine person enough, he may sing a song, but you won't learn it or remember it because he doesn't really mean for you to have it. He is just trying to get rid of you. Now they write it down or record it. I know carriers now who read off their notes when they make medicine. That person didn't know the medicine. That is why he is reading.

THE SPECIALIST

This category of *heles-hayv* also commands a unique respect in that this person's knowledge and serious lifestyle affects the well-being of the ceremonial ground and its people. The responsibility of the pure performance or rituals invoking powers for the well-being of the ground itself and its people is given into his hands by inheritance or selection. Unlike the other categories, this position is occupied by males only. The person has to be thoroughly versed in the ways of a particular ceremonial ground. He must know all rituals, medicines, and songs associated with that ground. He can be a carrier also and may perform extracurricularly to his duties for the ground.

Kērrv and Owalv

Nowadays people don't know the difference between *kērrv* and *owalv*. *Owalv* prescribes, tells you what is wrong. A good one, you don't tell them anything. He prescribes what you need, prophesies. *Owalv* is like a fortune teller. He can tell you what could take place tomorrow or ahead of time. He can tell you this is what you need because this is what is going to happen but he could also tell you what is wrong now. He can look back. He can tell past and future.

For example, let's say people have a lot of problems with certain things that are very unusual for them. There are people who want to know what happened, about when did it start, who did it? Those are the kind of questions they have for that *owalv*. Normally, the *owalv* won't tell them who did it because of what could take place. He may describe where that person lived, the area, or the direction or he may come out and say you know that person real well. It may be a relative somewhere too. He'll tell so much to them, but he wouldn't give that person's name away because there could be some killing going on. It can happen; it has happened. So he would explain, "alright, this is what happened, this was what was done to you, maybe eight months ago because of this. This is what shows up; it was over nothing," or whatever it was. He may say, "You all had a heck of a squabble at that time." And the *owalv* doesn't even have to be told anything in advance and yet he'll come out and say what happened.

Owalv can be a man or a woman. This is a gift. It is not necessary to be trained. This is something you are born with. You can not be trained to do this. This is a category. A main *heles-hayv* may not have this, but he might. A little child could make a statement that he shouldn't know about, like someone is going to come visit before it happened. If little things like that happened a couple of times, they would say, "This boy or girl has a special gift," and they would start watching the child closely. They always give them medicine to strengthen it anyway. They would instruct them not to say anything around people that are not within the family who knows about this. They would try to keep it a secret while he was growing up.

They do not want people bothering him to discourage him at a young age. Wait till he matures a little bit to where he can understand it himself. As a little child he wouldn't really understand what he has, until he grew up a little bit. He would not know how to handle it. If it is in his way, he might override it himself and eventually lose it. When he matures out, he could understand what he's got and would want to develop it. If you want him to be strong, you seek out somebody who can help him. They would get another medicine man to help him, strengthen him. You are working on his mind, also that he have a good clear mind. You are strengthening him. The medicine works on his motor system to keep his mind clear so he would be able to see things clearly, that it would come to him freely and that he would be able to concentrate when someone asked him a question. I don't know if there are any *owalv* left in the Creek Nation. I really don't. The ones I used to know, they're dead and gone, long time ago.

Now *kērrv*, we have got a few older ones around. *Kērrv* (one who knows) knows right now what is wrong. To make *kērrv* into a category is too much. He "knows" is an expression. But the person "knows" from experience. It is learned. Today most Mvskoke look at *kērrv* as a gift, but it was a person who had learned by experience. When I talk about "learned by experience," I'm talking about a child who has seen his mother or dad making medicine after seeing their clients and asking them questions about how the sickness is affecting them, how often it hurts, where it hurts, external or internal, if they are seeing a medical doctor, and so on. The child hears his mother or dad explain what he or she is going to be making for the client and how the medicine is to be used. I think you will now know how most *kērrv* come about. A young child who has watched and listened to the types of medicine being made will grow up knowing what causes certain sicknesses. I have cured sickness when the medical doctor didn't know what was wrong with a client. I was able to help because I was using my past experience of watching my grandmother and dad work. They had explained to me the symptoms of the sickness and its effect on a person and why certain sacred words and roots or leaves were being used for this certain sickness.

A main *heles-hayv* is usually gifted and thus he or she would likely have one or both of these gifts (*owalv* or *kērrv*), but a person can have one or both of these but not be a *heles-hayv*. But then, a *heles-hayv* "knows" what is wrong because of the training he received. He doesn't have to wait for lab tests. That is *kērrv*, "one who knows" what it is causing the problem.

Chapter Four

SELECTION OF
MEDICINE PEOPLE

THE SELECTION PROCESS

I'll tell you how my grandmother did and my dad. They knew my mother, her baby was going to be tested and if I should happen to be the one to be selected, my grandmother wanted to have an input. She delivered me but she wanted to have an input. So my dad was to make one medicine to see what kind of person I would be in fifty, sixty years. Would I keep our words sacred? And my grandmother made one medicine. Instead of my dad making both of them, she made one. And the medicine she made was for me to learn. That's why she worked with me more than Dad did, because she used that medicine over and over and over again for me to learn quickly and never forget the sacred words. My dad had the little gourds and he had already made a spoon out of a limb. No man-made things were used to even shape that little wooden spoon; he used a rock. He shaped it out with this sharp rock. The minute I was born, they gave me that medicine to see if I would take it. And they said, "You drank that medicine like you were thirsty for water. You went after that medicine." And they were satisfied; they knew that I would keep it sacred. And then my grandmother was the one who washed me down with that medicine that she had made. That was for me to learn quickly and never forget the medicine. And from that day on I guess she just kind of took over. She would keep working with me; she'd give me a bath with that medicine all the time until I learned everything I was supposed to learn. So within that span of time from when I was born to six years old, I knew the whole thing. When I was six and one-half years old, I was all ready to be initiated.[1]

LEARNING THE PLANTS

The first word I learned was heleswv (medicine). My grandmother said, "You didn't learn words like Mom and Dad like most children. The first word you learned was *heleswv*." But I think that everything that she'd touch that was medicine, she'd touch and then repeat, "this is medicine" until it was well etched in my mind, I guess. So when I could talk, that was the first word I said.

We didn't ask her questions. She didn't want you to ask her questions and she would tell you right quick. She'd say, "I'll tell you if I want you to know." And boy, that was it. That was our law at the house. But she was very patient, when I think back. She had to be to put up with me. I think what really stands out in my mind was the way she was teaching me about these plants in a way that I would never forget. She had to be real patient. Because I always remember when I got a little bigger, going with her. I would carry the thing that she was going to dig with. I thought it was a big deal and I'd walk in front of her. She said from the time that I could walk, she said that the grass was taller than I was, I'd lead the way, and off we'd go. When we went out to dig these roots we'd start from the farthest away to dig roots, then we'd start working our way back toward the house. And then I asked her, "Why do we have to always go so far to start digging for medicine? Why can't we just dig the first roots we come to and go on?" She said that one reason is that I was full of energy when we first started out. When I started to begin to tire out we were already back close to the house. We wouldn't have far to walk.

And the roots that we dug in the summertime, the leaves were very easy to identify. In the wintertime when all the leaves have fallen you have to know where they are in order to get them. She would dig all kind of roots, even old poison ivy roots. She would just bunch them all together and say, "We'll go wash them." She would lay them down and then try to figure out which ones were the medicine. She asked me to help her. I did it the way she did it before. I'd pick it up; I'd smell; I'd chew it. I think back and I chewed some of the poison ivy roots and never did catch anything. Why didn't I get sores in my mouth? She had ways. They use medicine anyway before they do these things. She had lots of roots, with very few of the medicine roots anyway. I'd go though the whole thing and find the medicine. She'd know how many were in there and I'd go through the whole thing until she was satisfied. I was about five. I could identify any of those roots that she could pick out, just by the smell and taste. I could tell her what root we had. I could tell her what it was used for. We could talk about one root. Then she would say, "What do you use it for?" That was the question I knew would follow. You didn't want her to ask you that so you would just tell her. Because you didn't want her telling you what it was used for because she would look down and then ask you something you are supposed to know. You beat her to it and tell her, "This is what we use it for," and whether we boil it or whether it could be taken just its natural way.

I asked her one time later, "How did you know that I would help?" And she said, "Kids like to play in dirt. I knew you'd help me dig." And then about washing them off, she said, "Kids like water. I knew you'd do it. I knew you'd wash them off."

LEARNING THE STORY

Now, the story about how this originated, she had a way. We'd sit out there on the porch and talk and she'd tell me the story of the origin of our medicine. I've always remembered there were at least three times in that story that she would throw something in that didn't relate to that story. In other words she would turn it around a little bit. I would break in and tell her that was not right and make her back up and tell it over. I was little, about four and one-half years old. I was pretty well on my way with it. At that time I could tell that story. And she'd back up and make the correction and we'd talk. Then she'd try to throw me off and I'd catch her again and tell her no, that's not right. Then about the third time she'd say, "If you know so much, then you tell the story." And then she'd let me tell the whole thing. When I think back, there was a purpose. That was her way of teaching me. That's why I said she had to be patient with me.

By the time you are six years old, you can tell the whole story back. It is a big, long story; it mentions every basic plant, how it began to grow. There are different plants, lots of other plants; it tells how each originated, how they began to grow. But you don't ever forget, that's the amazing thing. I like that. They condition you for that. That is why they give the chosen infant that bath so he will never forget. From the time I was born they were washing me down with medicine, washing my head with it.

My dad taught me about the plants too. I went out with him when I got a little older. My grandmother was the one who showed me the different ones when I was real little. I know Dad would mention some kind of sickness and ask me what kind of plant would you use and I would say well I would use this one here, or the bark of a certain tree. And he would want me to tell how I would use it, boil it or what. Dad had a different way than my grandmother.

BEING TESTED

I knew the plants and I knew the history of the medicine before I was ever initiated. That's when they really test you, just before you are initiated. The way my grandmother did it, she dug a lot of different plants. She had some old bitter roots, all kind of roots in there, and she had them all mixed together. And then she said, well, help her find which ones are the medicine roots. Nearly all of them had been used for some things, but she was looking for particular things, and I knew what she was talking about. And so I'd smell those things, I'd chew them and I'd throw them away. And then when I'd come on the one that she wanted I'd say, "Here, this is the medicine."

Another time, I went with my dad. He was going to sweat. I was little.

I had to take both hands to pick up a rock, so I had to be little. But, when I think back, the reason for what he did that day was to test me to really see if I was a firm believer. You have to believe in what you're doing, even when you are that little. But, anyway, he had the rocks ready for the sweat. The rock was already glowing red. And then he turned around and he told me, "Hand me the hottest rock." When I think back on it, I never did question him on how. Sometimes I think back to that day, I always remember getting that rock out. And then I handed it to him and I said, "This is the hottest rock." And then he just smiled. I've always remembered that smile. He was satisfied. Normally, they don't have to handle them. They've got a stick for them, but this particular time what he did was to see if I would obey and reach in there and get that rock. That was a test. But I think he had an idea that I would.

I probably will never do that again until I get ready to pass this down to the next one. That child that you're bringing up, you have him well protected. That's why I wasn't afraid of that rock and it didn't burn me. Because he had already done things, what we call cooling that flame off, where we could handle that. And so, if I ever pass this down, I'll do the same thing. And the child will not even be afraid to handle that because you teach them so much that they are well conditioned. They'll automatically do it. When the child picks it up it never burns him anyway, because you take care of that part for him. I didn't hesitate. He was just seeing if I would obey and do it. I didn't question. I went in there, got one rock out and said, "This is the hottest rock." My first taste of sweat. And after that I didn't sweat with him. He said, "You have to get your own." Oh, I used to go down there with him all the time. I'd get the wood for him, but I never took sweat with him. I wasn't allowed to after the first one. He showed me what was expected of me to do and the sacred words to use for a sweat and why.

All of this medicine we're talking about, they teach you this over and over again that you're conditioned for just about anything you talk about or do; you never question it. All you know is that you're gonna do it. You never say, "Huh? why?" You don't ask questions; you just carry it through. And I think that's one of the most important tests, what kind of person you'll be, whether you'll obey them. If you didn't obey your parents at that age, then you might misuse your medicine later on in life. You'll be hard-headed. So I think they were really testing you to see if you would carry this through. They had to know. They had to know because of what they were getting ready to give you. Like I've said before, they give you one good with one bad. And they have to know who someday will have all these powers to do certain things.

INITIATION

By the age of six I knew the basic roots that we would always use regularly. We had a lot of other plants, leaves and bark from different trees, that were learned later on. You had to know the basic roots first. The key to the whole thing was that you know the history. It wasn't so much knowing the roots. They want you to know that, but that wasn't the important thing. The important thing was that you had to know the origin of your medicine before you were ever initiated. That was the reason that they harped on it.

My grandmother initiated me when I was around six and one-half years old.[2] She had all the medicine made that she was going to use that day. We went to the water, running water, a stream. I was facing east. She had a gourd, the biggest size that she could find. And she had gotten ready. She had some red roots in there and then she had a small gourd, a little bitty one, that she dipped into the other one. She had four different rocks. I won't mention them all; one of them I will. She handed me a rock and then she said this, "That you will have the power to heal the sick." And then she handed it to me and told me, "Bury it in the bottom of that stream there. Embed it in the water."

I went under and I put that little rock in that water. And then when I came up she poured that medicine on me. And then she gave me another one and she described what other things I had the power to do. And each time I'd come up she poured that medicine on me. And after the fourth one she was through. I remember she turned around facing back east, and she said that she had carried out the thing that she was supposed to do. She carried out the instruction that day. She said, "He has the power. All the power is within this little man. Someday he'll have to carry out all things medicine people have been instructed to do." And then, I always remember she held that gourd up, she raised it up and that old gourd popped. I mean just like somebody was slamming it against a wall. And you know how they'll shatter, just like that. It popped and scattered everywhere. She just threw that in the water like it was nothing. And then she turned around and looked at me. She said, "This is your day," and went back home and left me down there, standing there. So I walked out of the stream and came up on the bank. I saw her going and that was very unusual; she never left me down there by myself. I was too little. I started to go—that's when I heard that voice that said, "Come here." I mean, loud, clear. I never did get scared. I just walked toward where the voice came from, I guess about, maybe fifteen, twenty yards; then I stopped. I didn't see anybody. There were some trees there, but there was nobody behind them. So I started to turn around and go back toward the house.

When I started to turn around and was a little farther off, it said, "Come over *here*." Then I came upon a rock there, a big flat rock, and I stopped right at the foot of that rock. And then I looked and right in the middle of that rock, there was a little cylinder about the size of a bowl, about five or six inches deep. I mean, beautifully cut, and evenly cut. If you saw it today you'd say it looked like they did that with a machine because it was beautifully cut. Right in the middle of that big rock there were the red roots and the water, the medicine. I jumped up on that rock and I looked down and it was there. It caught my eye. I reached in there, I took that root out and I chewed on it and put it back. And then the voice said, "Wash with it." My hand went down in there and I just washed my head. When you say "Wash with it" that usually means just soak your head, and I did that. When that last voice was heard, that was it. I got off that rock, and I don't know why, but I jumped off and I turned around; I don't know why. Then right in the middle of that rock I could hear the cracking of that rock. You could hear popping. And the whole thing split right in the middle. It broke in two and the medicine that was in there just spilled all out. And when I think back to that day, everything that we used in initiations was only used one time and then it was destroyed. Like that gourd I told about, it was destroyed. It wasn't done by my grandmother and that rock wasn't done by anybody else. But that son of a gun, it cracked right down the middle. And then after that happened, I played in the water a little bit and went on home. Even today I still call it "mystery rock," and I've always said I'll take a picture. I go down there and sit down on it, but I've never done it yet. I have a camera with me, but I still have never taken a picture. It's still there. One of these days, I've said, I'll cut off the piece with the cylinder. There is a pretty good size piece left on there. Maybe I'll take out the piece with the cylinder and square it and keep it. But maybe it wasn't meant for me to keep.

When my dad initiated me, it was kind of comical in a way. It was wintertime. We went down to the water. I didn't walk in the water like I did with my grandmother. It was in the summertime when she walked right in there and I followed her. She found the deepest part. My dad didn't do it that way. He went to the water with me. It was a flat rock and the water was running right through, just a few feet from the top of that rock. And then I saw that there was ice on top of that water. And I'm supposed to get in that water with that ice on there, you see. So, I kneeled down and I cracked that ice and then I stuck my hand in there. That water was cold. I got up and I told my dad, "I don't want to be a medicine man." And that made him mad. He told me it wasn't cold. He told me to feel it. He said, "The water's not cold." I turned around and when I did that he shoved me and into the water I went. Everything my grandmother did, he did the same thing. Well, he said it in different words. The wording was his. Then when I got through, I raised up to get out and that cold wind hit. It was cold. I went back into the water up to my mouth, because it was warm. I wouldn't get out of there. And that made Dad mad, too. I've always remembered he said, "I told you to get out of that water." And I wouldn't do it. He really got mad. He jumped in that water. He grabbed me by the seat of my pants and, boy, he walked straight across to the other bank and took me home. He was walking fast, too. I used to tease him about that. I said, "Dad, I made you get in that water with me, too." A few things we just teased each other about; that is one of the things that always stands out in my mind.

LEARNING THE WORDS

Right after initiation, they could start giving you the words to the songs.[3] Before that no songs are given out. You can hear them; you can listen to them; you could learn them. They don't teach you, but you could pick it up. You can sing; you know what they're saying. But, directly, they do not start singing to you until after initiation. And then, that's when they really start putting it in you. When they get ready to do a chant, when they're going to give you some words to some of those songs, they prepare you first. Wash your face with the medicine. They also prepare themselves and the reason is so that your mind is ready to receive and she's ready to give or he's ready to give. And they sit down. They'll go through each medicine chant very slowly. They say them one by one. The chants are never sung while being taught. You just go through the words. Go through the whole words. And the amazing thing about it is you can hear it one time and you can say the whole thing, all of it, back to them. It's almost unbelievable sometimes when you just sit around and think in the white man's way. How can anybody pick that up? But this is what they prepare you for from a baby on up, so that you can hear it once and not forget it.

My grandmother would get through with me and she'd tell me to repeat. They don't teach a lot of them at one time, maybe two or three. I would sit there, and let the whole thing go through my mind, just what she said. I mean, it was just like listening to a radio. You sat there; you could hear her say all the things that she said, over in your mind. After she's already been through it, in the back of your mind you can still hear the same thing. And then you turn right around, and you can repeat words like you're reading them off a paper, almost seeing the words. It's there. And you'd get through and she'd smile, and then she'd say, "Well, I'm going to tell you another one." Then she'd go through the whole thing.

And then when you'd get through with three of them, she'd say, "I want to hear all three of them. I want to hear the middle one, then the first one, and the last one." It would never be in the same order.

My dad used to ask to hear them too. We'd be talking about other things, and all at once he'd say to sing certain things. He wanted you to hit it right there without even thinking about it. You could be sitting around eating and they'd say, "I want to hear earache or spider bite words." Just like that. You'd stop eating and, boy, you'd just rattle it back to them, and then you'd get back to eating. I mean they're just liable to ask you to say certain medicine words any time. You're supposed to know it. All they did was just smile, no words. They didn't say, "That's a good boy" or anything. They just smiled and that was it. Unique way of teaching. Good. I think the key to the whole thing is preparing you when you're little, when you're not supposed to forget. When I got a little older, I once asked my grandmother, "Why don't you do that to me where I can learn in school?" She said, "This is a different school you're going to. This is my school."

See, the story that they were telling back then was the same story, from both sides. And the thing about it is the chants are different. Her chants are entirely different from my dad's and yet they are for the same purpose; the same type of roots, you use them the same. Everything is the same except the words—the chants are altogether different.[4]

FINDING THE TUNES

Even in visions you're given the words. No song, just the words. When my grandmother went through the song that she had, she just said the words. What you do is that when you go out, you fast. Anytime that you are going to go out and do a medicine and you are going to go out in the woods by yourself, normally you fast; it's just almost a routine. When you're out there you go for a purpose, go to fulfill something, and everything falls into place. You listen to the sound of nature, the rustling of the leaves in the trees when the wind's blowing, the pitch of that wind. You listen to that and then add the sound to the words. You now have a tune to that song. Not all of the tunes to any of the songs that you have are one and the same. It's hard to explain. It's just that the medicine people do what is suited for them.

You don't use the same tune to each medicine even if it is almost the same in a way. But you always make that tune appropriate to the words in the song. You're tuned to certain words, you know. Out in the woods you just go, you sit. You listen and then it'll start coming to you. In a little bit you can have a tune to a song and you can go through that, and then the chant has a pretty tune to its words.

Once you put a tune to it, it'll stay with you. Let's say that you go out, and you've got words, and you listen, and the sounds that you hear, you then put them into a tune, with the words you have, and you go through that. Once you go through that one time, there's a tune to that. You'll always use that. It's kind of strange—it just never goes off, it's there. It's like recording and then you stick it back into the machine and you listen to it again, and it'll repeat itself. It's about the same thing. Once you put a tune to it it'll always be there. It's there.

I used to sit on the edge of a rock with my feet dangling, just sit there, swinging away, and then I'd be singing away. It just comes to you left and right. It's strange the way it happens. I'd come home and I'd be singing. They'd get after me, too. I would get out on the porch and then I'd put a tune with the words. I had such little short legs, and the porch was high back then to me. They said I'd sit there with my feet dangling and I'd be just singing away. My grandmother told me to cut that out—there was no monkey business. But I was proud I had learned something; I could put a tune to it. So I wanted to sing that song. I would. I'd sit out there and I wouldn't pay attention. But I always stopped, too. My grandma said, "You'd be out there. If anybody else tried to sneak up on you," she said, "listen to what you were singing, you'd quit, and you'd just jump off and you'd start playing; go out there and start playing." She said, "You'd just sit out there and dangle your feet back and forth, you'd be just singing away." I must've been a mean little boy then, hard head, especially after I learned to put a tune to one of them. She said, "That's when you opened up, too. You were just singing away."

There was one song that she always teased me about. At the end it has a kind of a sound of a drum; that's the way you wind it down. But I'd come on the porch and I was winding it up. She said I'd stomp my feet. "You'd stomp your feet as you were ending that song, and then you'd come right in like nothing happened." She said, "I watched you, you'd be singing away and then you'd get to the end of the song and then you had to stomp your feet and then come on in. You'd come through there like you owned the world. You'd stomp your feet, wind up your song, and come right on through like you owned the world." Those were the good old days.

ACQUIRING A MEDICINE STICK

The medicine stick is the main tool of all medicine people in Mvskoke culture.[5] The length or size of the stick used is up to the person using it. The chant or words are sung from one end of the stick going through and out the other end. After each song is sung, the medicine man blows into the stick to push the words through into the water, which is now being mixed with medicine roots and words to complete making the medicine.

The one who is teaching you will always give you their medicine stick, the one that they use the most. They'll give you one of theirs. And then when you get your own, the one that they have given you is retired, will never be used again. They'll give you that medicine stick any time, once you learn your words. They'll present it to you. You fast; they'll give you a bath with the medicine, and then they'll hand it to you. They'll say, "This is yours. This is your tool. Keep it sacred. Until you get yours, you use this until you get your own. When you get your own, you will retire this stick never to be used again." After they give you theirs, they have got one all ready to go; so they give you theirs and then they get that new one out.

There is a process for selecting your medicine stick that nobody knows about. In our tribe, they don't even know. You fast. The person fasts to get himself ready. He prepares himself and then he goes out and he looks for the medicine stick. He'll select the one that he wants, then he'll tie it. He'll tie that certain plant with a red cloth or something red. Lots of times a plant is found when it's dry ground, but that medicine stick, the reed there, will never be cut until it is standing in running water. In other words, they are water reeds. And as long as there's no water running, even if it's wet around the stick, it's never touched until a good rain comes and the water is running and that plant is in that water, the running water. That'll be the only time that he'll ever cut that water reed. When the water's running, it's purified by that water. Then you really go to work to purify that stick. You retire those others. The ones that were given to you will never be used again. You put a feather on each end of it to cap it off. The words will never go in one end or out the other end. Just cap it off. You do the same process of purification when you retire a stick that you do when you prepare a newly cut one. All these are prepared. You clean it. You sprinkle it down and it cleans the whole thing. You purify it and then you cap it off with feathers on each end. We prefer eagle feathers if we have them. We use a lot of hawk feathers. Any chance we get to use an eagle feather, we use it. Being from a bird clan like I am, we're authorized to use any feather, any bird. Then you put the stick away. I've got two old sticks at home. They'll always be there, I guess.

MAKING MEDICINE FOR THE FIRST TIME

This man was a medicine man, ceremonial ground medicine man. But he had an earache, and there's not too much you can do with an earache. My grandmother was over there at his mother's side house. So he came down there and wanted my grandmother to doctor. He said he had not slept for a couple of nights and had a bad earache. He said, "I can't sleep." My grandmother, she looked down at me and said, "You do it. You help him. This is what I prepared you for. You're ready. You do it." Just like that, out of the blue. And from that day I've always appreciated that man because he never said no or anything. He smiled. He looked down at me and he knew my grandmother. He knew that she had taught me. So he believed in me also. When I think back, he had to let me do it.

But this guy was so tall there was no way I could reach his head, so I went around one side. I went round and round him, trying to figure out how I was going to reach his head to help him. But he was laughing; he had a smile. Finally he knelt down for me. I've always remembered that. He knelt down. That was the first medicine I ever made, and that was for another medicine man. I've always had a lot of respect for him because he believed in me enough to let me do it. But my grandmother, the way she brought me up, she knew that I was ready. I had to be ready before I was initiated, but then she never hesitated once. She just looked down; she said, "You help him." Just like that. "You help him." I was prepared; she said, "You're ready." And I never did question that, either. My question was, "How do I reach this man's head? He's too tall."

HELP FROM TEACHERS

One thing they teach you, they'll tell you over and over, is that you will never forget. But if there are times that some things are bothering you, how to treat a person, for example, and you are trying to figure out the best way and the quickest way to treat a person, Dad always said, "We're by you. We'll be there. When you need help, you'll hear a voice. You need help, we'll be there."[6] For example, if I were to lie down, and I was thinking of one of the longer songs I haven't used in a long time, I'd go to sleep. Then during the night, if it's Dad's song or my grandmother's song—it doesn't matter which—I'd hear the same voice again. It'll go through the whole thing for me in my sleep. And when I get up next morning it's just like it's fresh on my mind. That's what they were talking about. "We'll be there when you think you have a problem with these things. We don't ever forget. We may be a little slow. You may have to sit there maybe a little bit to make sure that you get the words all right."

And there were times that I was hesitant about which medicine I would use for certain sicknesses. And then I would decide and I would go to bed and plan to make it the next morning. Then at night my grandmother would say, "Why don't you do it this way? Use this song." She'd sing the whole thing over and then she'd say, "This is what you need to use."

You could hear her like she was sitting there talking. Next day, I would get up and think, "I could cut out a lot of things by doing it the way she mentioned. That'll get the whole job done. If I had used my own idea, I might have had to use two songs for this thing. Her way I can use one." That's what I mean. They're there when you need them. I've heard her voice, I've heard Dad's voice, "Use this. It'll be the quickest way to get to the point, to get this thing done right. Use this song; use these roots. It'll be a lot faster than the way you want to do it." These people were experienced. I've got experience, too, but they get their two cents' worth in every once in a while.

They never leave.

Chapter Five

MEMORIES OF CHILDHOOD
IN A MEDICINE FAMILY

I have always remembered the good times when I was a child. These are stories about my grandmother and my dad and the medicine.

HEALING THE COUSIN

One day a cousin and I were playing in a tree, acting like monkeys in the tree. But there was a little chicken pinned on the south side of that tree where we had an enclosure with a big fence, hog wire. The little chicken got caught in that wire. I was climbing down the tree to go around to the gate to free that little chicken, and my cousin decided he was going to beat me over, do it first, so he hung on a limb across that fence and he jumped. There were some dead limbs. When he jumped, one of the limbs went through his pants and into his leg and hit a vein. We had a lot of people at the house at that time. They picked him up. They took him and laid him on the porch. We didn't have a telephone, but our neighbor did. They went over to the neighbor's house and called a doctor, an old, old man. The doctor came down there in a Model A. They had to remove some of my cousin's pants. They cut his pants where you could see the stick sticking out of his leg. The doctor came down there, he looked at it a while, and he said, "You'll have to bring him up to my place to work on it." But he made a mistake. He pulled that little stick out, and boy, the blood squirted out like a stream. It shot out. That shook the doctor up. He said, "Hurry and load him up 'cause he'll bleed to death." That shook him up.

In the meantime, my dad had been hunting and he was just getting back to the house. There was a trail there; he came back up and a lot of them ran to meet him to tell him what was wrong. He came around the corner and said, "What's all this fuss about?" That old doctor who was shook up was trying to bandage my cousin, get the pressure point. Dad went over and he looked at it. My uncle had his thumb on there while that old man was wrapping it up. Dad told him, "Move your hand." I always remember that. Slapped his hand and told him to move it. And he looked at it. That blood came back out. Dad said, "That's nothing." And so he turned around and he walked back behind the house. On the north side where we were, there was a fence there, but he stepped over that fence. Then he came back with a little ball of dirt just a little bit bigger than a marble. He came back and he told the doctor, "Move your hand," again. And he took that little roll of dirt. He put it on there for just a little. I'm not talking about five or six minutes; he just held it there a while. I would say probably about a minute or two. That was about all. And then he just took that dirt, moved that dirt, and there wasn't a drop of blood coming out.

And that old doctor, he stood there; he shook his head and said, "You don't need me. You've got all the help you need right here." And that's when I told my dad, "Dad, I want to be just like you. I want to be just as good as you." So, when I think back then, I wanted to be like him, I wanted to be as strong because I knew he was good.

GETTING TO TOWN THE FAST WAY

There was a dirt road that went west or north (forked road), about a half mile from where I lived. There used to be a row of mailboxes at that corner. That used to be the mail route and still is, but back then the mail carriers didn't go down to the bottom to deliver our mail to us like they do now. Anyway, at the forked road where all these mailboxes were, there was a full-grown peach tree that provided a good shade and that was where most of the Indians would sit and wait for the mailman or wait for someone to give them a ride into town. During the hot, summer Saturdays when my dad would take me to town to let me eat and go to a movie, this was where Dad and I would sit and wait for a ride. There were times we would be walking and people would stop for us and offer us a ride and we would ride with them. And there were times when Dad would thank them and say, "We're going to walk." He meant both of us were going to walk all the way to town on that day, but what the heck, it was only nine and a half miles to town. There were times he would let me ride with some people we knew after telling me where we would meet. Dad would say to me, "Go ahead and ride with them. I'll be up there in a little while. Go ahead and ride." So, I'd get in. The car wouldn't make a stop either on the way to town, and we'd leave him right under that tree. My uncle and his wife would let me ride with them, never making a stop on the way to town and leaving my dad standing under the shade tree.

This is the most interesting part of my story, and some of the people talk about it today. As you got into the town you would have to cross the railroad tracks to go up the main street. Just as you crossed the tracks there was a hotel on the south side of the street and a cafe on the north side. Across the street, to the west side of the hotel, was a grocery store where my dad traded. There was some shade there so many of the Indians would stand around, talk, and visit with each other. Coming into town, I

would be sitting back there in the pickup enjoying myself; Susie, my uncle's
wife, used to tap on the back window of the pickup and point toward the
grocery store. My dad would be standing in the shade talking to some of
his friends that were there. We just left him back at the forked road. He
was standing under the tree by the mailboxes when we left him and yet
he beat us to town. Now, that was something. But there are ways that
we travel. That is what he was doing. An Indian, even of another tribe,
would know what I am saying, but non-Indians, it would be hard for them
to understand. But there are ways; it can be done. I don't know if you
want to call it "speed travel," I don't know what. He did his own thing to
move himself from this place to that place, and he was there ahead of us.
He used medicine. He used what he was taught by my great grandfather,
Jackson Lewis. Without riding with us, he beat us there. Because that is
what he did; it can be done. He just traveled from one place to another
his own way. Every once in a while he did that. That's what I mean. He
was that good.

   If we were going to walk, he would give me a little old root and say,
"Here, chew this." He walked fast too; Dad walked fast. I never did get
tired. People would stop to give us a ride. He'd say, "No, we'll walk." I'd
say, "Dad, I want to ride." But he'd say, "No, we are going to walk." But I
never did get tired. And I would walk. I walked nine and a half miles and
stayed up with him. Now you couldn't get me to walk a mile.

BECOMING INVISIBLE

There were some things Dad would do often, but his favorite thing was
becoming invisible. I would visit him frequently at the church ground
where he lived then in a camp house. There were times he wouldn't be
home and his dog would be gone, which indicated to me that he was close
by. The first place I would look was toward a trail that goes around a
pond and into the woods. I would sit and wait on him with my eyes on
the trail, hoping to see him or his dog. I would really be looking for the
dog, because his dog stayed with him all the time no matter where he went
and always walked in front of him. Suddenly, out came the little dog from
the woods and into the clearing; I knew Dad was on his way back home.
I would continue looking but there was no movement out there, nothing
that I could see. I knew he was close but I didn't know where he was. His
dog was always a giveaway that he was close by and his dog had come
back into the church yard and almost back to the camp house. I would
continue watching his dog till it lay down; now I knew Dad was back, but
I couldn't see him so I would look around some more for him, even call
out to him. And I turned back around; he would be standing right beside

me. He had gone for a walk and come back unseen. He was back on the church ground and back to the camp house all this time. He wasn't there and he was there. I would tease and joke with him about this. I knew his answer but I would always say to him, "Up to your tricks again, Dad?" He just laughed and said, "No, just practicing," and we both laughed.

Dad didn't like me to do something like that to him, though. I did pull a few tricks on him, but I sure got chewed out and he wouldn't ask me if I was practicing either. He had his favorite lawn chair in the shade; so one time when he was not there, I sat down after turning the chair toward the direction he would be coming. Out of the woods and into the clearing I saw him taking his time coming by the water and following his favorite trail, going around the pond and back into the church yard. Being tired from his walk, he walked up to his lawn chair, put his hand on the chair's arm, and sat down on my lap. I gave him a shove and said, "Get off me, Dad!" He jumped off my lap and started chewing me out. He had his cane still in his hand and I thought he was going to hit me with it. He told me to never do that to him again. Pointing his finger at me, he said, "Don't ever pull that on me again. I have a bad heart." Dad gave me a good scolding, but never did ask me if I was practicing.

This is just one of the minor things we do, not to be funny but to bring out some old teaching. It is to keep our words fresh and strong at all times in case there is ever a need for them. I may never have to use them, but just in case, I will be ready.

UNDERSTANDING TORNADOES

I was over visiting my dad at the church ground and we were sitting under a small shade tree. He said, "Son, we're going to have a bad weather." I answered, "Yeah, looks like we're going to have a heck of a storm and I have a bad feeling about this one." It wasn't too long a wait before the sky got dark with rain clouds and we were hearing a loud roaring sound that was getting closer. That was making me feel uneasy because I'd heard that sound before. Before a tornado ever touches down you usually hear its loud roaring sound. I said to Dad, "You know, a high wind is coming." He answered, "I know it; I've been expecting it for a few days now." The sound in the air was getting louder and I knew that a tornado was in the air; sooner or later it would touch down somewhere nearby.

He caught me looking at the cellar. He said, "No, we're going to sit right here. Don't worry about it. We'll stay right here." The sound of a roar was getting to me so I said to Dad, "Don't you think we ought to go to the cellar?" He answered with anger in his voice, "No, we'll stay right here." He knew I wasn't in total agreement with him, so he said, "If you want to go to the cellar, you can." I said, "Dad, if you don't go, I sure won't go either." I don't think I could forgive myself if I had run out on him that day when he needed me to believe him and the medicine he used getting ready for this storm.

My dad's camp house is located on the northeast corner of our church ground. There is a little shed right close that we built many years ago to store our tools. It is right close to the camp house and it was ready to blow over. Right beside the shed were two full-grown peach trees. I would say we were sitting less than fifty feet from the shed and peach trees. Suddenly, the tornado came down out of the sky and it touched the ground and it took one of the peach trees up and it was gone. The tree disappeared. The little shed we had was so old, I believe you could have leaned against it hard and it would have fallen over; yet not one board came off that shed, nothing. His camp house roof shingles were so old and brittle that the roof could easily have been ripped apart with just a high wind blowing, but not one shingle came off.

Just imagine you are watching a tornado coming out of the sky and pulling up one peach tree out of two that were standing and not ever hurting that one tree left standing. You are sitting and watching as a tree disappears in a second. Dad never did make a move to take shelter. I didn't either; maybe I was too scared to move. Dad was prepared for this storm; I wasn't. He was well prepared ahead of time before I ever got over to his place.

That was just another experience for me to witness what my dad could do. I will always remember his words on that day when he said, "I'm going to stay here; if you want to go to the cellar, you can." I answered, "If you won't go, I'm not going to run either." I sat with my dad as we watched a tornado pull a peach tree up so close to the shed and never do any damage to camp house or shed. It was almost unbelievable. That was a good experience that I had with my dad, sitting together, being shown what our medicine people can do with Mother Nature. I have seen tornados before. I almost got caught in one before, so I know what they can do. I have seen them take big trees down, snap them up out of the ground like they were nothing, and yet it never did blow one shingle off my dad's house.

CURING SNAKEBITE

Dad and I went to look for plants down near Sallisaw where the rocky places are. He was well prepared. We both were, but the thing about it was that he didn't hear the snake. It was right close. It bit Dad. Where Dad got bit, it bled itself out. I have always remembered. It bled. And that rattler that bit Dad was curled back up. Do you know that old snake died while we were still there? That rattlesnake, it never did uncoil. That's why I said Dad was good. There were some miracles that I saw him do. He was very good. That old snake never did move after it curled back to strike again. Dad walked a little way. He sat down on a little flat rock. He untied his shoe, took his sock off, and rolled his pants leg up. It got him, oh, not too high up. He said, "We'll sit a little bit." So we just sat there a little bit and I watched. It started bleeding. Just like if you cut around where you have been bit, it started bleeding like that. Blood went down toward his foot. It bled for a little while and all at once it quit. And Dad wiped it off and put his sock and shoe back on and tied his shoe, and he rose and said, "Let's go." And then he went over and kicked that old rattler over. That thing was dead. I kicked it too. I wanted to make sure that it was dead. It was dead. But Dad never even thought one thing about it—never even gave it a second thought. I thought about it though. I remember shaking my head, and I thought, "Dad's good. He is good." You have to see things that I've seen. That is why I have said, "They've got some powerful people." Not just my grandma and my dad. Those others, they were good. I mentioned that time he stopped my cousin bleeding. That snake never did uncoil again. They were good. That's why I say we prepared when we went out and did these things. That is why we are not afraid of anything.

THE CHICKENS ON THE BUS

Let me tell you a story that happened to me and my grandmother. We went to McAlester to see some people down there. We rode a bus. They picked us up and then she made medicine for those people. And when we got ready to come back, they decided to give her some chickens and a rooster. But we were going to ride a bus, so they put them all in a box. They tied up the box and normally I don't think you're allowed to carry those things on a bus, but they let her. They didn't say anything. So we got on the bus and she had the box in her hand, and we sat down.

We got over there by Checotah, and somehow the chickens got loose. I think we had about four hens and a rooster in there. It wasn't all that big a box, either. Small box. Somehow it opened up and they got loose and when they got loose they were flying everywhere. The bus driver pulled off to the side of the road and the chase was on. People were grabbing for the chickens. The rooster was the one that gave them a bad time. That part was kind of comical because of everybody chasing chickens on the bus. They were flying everywhere. You'd touch them, and they'd fly. The driver finally caught that old rooster and they put him in the box. Finally we caught them all and boxed them back up and came on home.

Now, that was a good experience for me. You don't chase chickens on a bus, but we did that day. Those chickens were something the people she made medicine for gave her in appreciation of what she had done. That was a little extra they gave her. I think they gave her a little bit of money, too. But they didn't think they were giving her enough. They appreciated her help so much that they wanted to give her some extra things. "Four hens and a rooster would really be nice."

PLAYING WITH THE "BALL"

There was one thing that my grandma used to do every so often. There used to be an old road that went through right by our front yard. Not too far from the house there used to be a barn. But there used to be a light—oh, about the size of a little baseball—that would pop up at night and it would move around. It was usually off the ground, I would say about three feet. It wasn't too far off the ground. There is no name for it in English. I've heard a lot of explanations, but it is a different type of energy that nobody has ever really got their hands on. But some of the white people have seen it too, because I've heard them talk about it. I've heard a lot of Indians talk about it.

Every once in a while it would move around and my grandmother used to say, "You want to play? Let's play with that ball." And then she would go in the house, she would fix medicine, she would come back out, we would wash with it. We would wash our faces and we would sit out on the porch. And we would point at it. And then we would move our hands this way. That old ball would go that way. And then she would go the other way with her arms and the ball would move the other way. We would control that little red ball out there. Any way that our hands went, that thing followed it. We would play with it for a while and then we would get tired of it and we would double up our fists, and then we would open our hands up fast and that thing would just pop. You've seen how firecrackers whenever they explode they make a little spark? That thing would do that and then just disappear.

She was that good. We didn't see that fire too often. But when we did, while we were sitting out there and we would see it, she would say, "Let's play with that ball." She used to call it a ball. Our hand would go one direction and that thing would follow and then all at once we would just jerk our hand and that thing would stay up with us. She would do it this way and then I would do it that way—in other words, we were trying to outguess each other. She would go that way and then I would take it away from her and I would jerk it back the other way, and so she would go and she would do it this way and I would do it that way, and that little ball just followed. And then we would get tired of it and she would say, "Let's let it go." Just like that we would double up our fists and then we would open them up like we were throwing it away, and then all at once that thing would just disappear. Both fists. We would be facing toward it and we would stop it in midair, like we were throwing it away, and we would open up our hands and it would disappear, just pop and it was gone. She was that good. She could control things.

I never thought too much about that. A lot of things that happened were almost immaterial to me because you see a lot of things and it is nothing important, really. To me it isn't. You grow up around our culture and you see these things all the time. And it is kind of routine, nothing to get excited about. But other people, now, it is really something to them. But to me it isn't. It is really nothing. I guess that is what we are trying to bring out.

THE LAST GATHERING

I've always called it the last gathering of the most powerful Mvskoke medicine people. I had already been initiated, so it was probably in the fall of 1940. They had set a date. And they all gathered at the house. They had a big container of medicine right in the middle of the floor. They would dip it out, then they'd go out and they'd wash their faces, and then they'd sit down and do all their talk. The last gathering there, they were gathering to talk about the techniques that they had used in the past and talking about the people that had already passed on and what was left. And they were also talking about how they were on the verge of losing all this. And I think a lot of them didn't have a replacement, that's what they were talking about—that they had not found a replacement for them if anything should happen to them. That was the end of that. There were some words passed back and forth and the techniques that they used. Mostly the techniques.

See, each one has got different songs, even though they do the same thing. So, they would go out and they'd talk about the techniques and there are certain roots that you can use as a substitute for another one. Which one they used the most—those things were talked about. And they took a break and then they were standing outside on the porch. One little short man was teasing this tall guy. He pointed out a bent little tree, a young sapling out there, and he was telling this tall one, "You're beginning to look like that tree, you know. You're humped over." He was teasing about the other man getting old. "You're beginning to look like that little tree over there."

So, they teased each other awhile and then some of them smoked, some of them chewed nearly all day. They came back and washed their mouths, spit all this out, then they went back into the house to sit down to do their talk. I've always remembered the sad look on their faces before they left that day because they knew that this was the last gathering. They knew that, when they got ready to go. I remember tears in my grandmother's eyes; they were coming down her cheeks. I didn't really understand at that time, why she was crying. It wasn't crying out, just tears rolling down. I remember crying. It wasn't for me, it was for her because I saw her hurt. But they all came outside and just before they left, another little short one—it wasn't the same one that had been teasing before—said, "Let's go talk to that tree." And nothing was said; they all went out to that tree and they put their hands on that tree.

I was crowding in between legs and getting up in there, too. Little kids want to do what the older people do. They put their hands up on that tree. And this little tree was so bent over that one limb was on the ground. It was just an ugly little tree, sickly little thing. They put their hand on that tree. All of them were all saying the same thing. They were telling that tree to stand tall and straight. And the little tree and limb popped and cracked upward as if it was reaching for our Creator. They told the limb to get off the ground and point toward the Creator, as if it were reaching for the Creator. And while they had their hands on that little old tree, you could hear it popping. You could actually hear it snapping. From being bent over, while they were still standing there with their hands on it, it slowly stood straight up. And the limb that was down there on the ground, they were bracing it up. It came up into a beautiful tree.

And that's why I'm saying these were powerful people. That was a day that they were talking about Jackson Lewis. That's the first time I ever heard Jackson Lewis's name, it would stay with me the rest of my life—but they were talking about him. "We lost some good people. We lost some powerful medicine men, medicine women." One man asked my grandmother, "Who do you think was the most powerful medicine person of all?" And she hesitated; I've always remembered that. She said, "I'll answer that." She said, "This is my own opinion." I remember her repeating that twice, "This is my own opinion. We've lost some good people, powerful people. There's very few of us left." She knew they were powerful, too. "There's very few of us left, but," she said, "this is my own opinion. Jackson Lewis stood above us all." And every one of them agreed to it. I remember them shaking their heads—that means that's true. That's what they were saying.

After I got older, that's what always made me think back about my great grandfather. What did he do so great that they looked up to him as most powerful—yet I witnessed something that they did that was very powerful. I saw them make that tree stand up straight. I was there. And yet they said Jackson Lewis stood above them all. What did he do so great that they looked up to him as being the greatest of all? And even today I'm always looking for an answer. What could he have done that made him so great? I'll never know the answer, but I saw what they did and I know they were powerful. But when you look up to somebody, he had to do something so great, so powerful that they thought he was the top. That he stood above them all. Jackson Lewis was a name that would stay with me the rest of my life. At that time it meant nothing. I didn't know Jackson Lewis. That was the first time I ever heard that name.

But they all agreed. My dad was there. He agreed that day. Maybe he was a little partial, I don't know. But those others didn't have to be. My grandmother didn't have to be that way. My grandmother was pretty darn powerful. They looked up to her, too. That's why they came down there to her house a lot. That day I saw a miracle happen. I still say they were the most powerful people that I would ever see. I got to witness that last gathering of the most powerful people. There were eight of them; two were women. They were great. Even till today I've always wondered, "Who were they?" I knew them, but I never knew them by their names. I always called them "Uncle." In fact there were no name references, just "Uncle" or "Grandpa." I called the women "Grandma." I didn't call them by their names. It was respect.

That tree, no matter where I'd been, when I got back home, I always went to that tree. Nobody ever knew why. Nobody ever knew. No matter where I'd been that's the first stop that I would make when I got back home, I would go out there and I'd stand and look at it. I once watched that little thing straighten up and it had grown to be a big tree. I saw the powerful people talk to this tree at one time. And the tree, it obeyed too. That's something that can't be forgotten. That's why that plant had to obey. In the story of the origin of our medicine, the plants have said, "You carry your end of our bargain and we'll carry ours. We'll meet you halfway." The plants would listen. That day that tree listened. One time I came back to visit and the tree no longer was there. My uncle had made a firewood out of it. I was really hurt when I came back and it was gone. That tree was just a reminder that I had witnessed something that nobody will ever witness again. It'll never happen again. But I was there. And I always think about my great grandfather. What did he do? It'll probably haunt me the rest of my life, wanting to find out why. Why, or how, was he so great?

FIRST ENCOUNTER WITH THE LITTLE PEOPLE

There is a flat rock down by the water in the woods there, near the house. I used to lie down on it and fish. Right on the west side of that there was a divot—a big tree had fallen all the way across the creek. I had gone fishing. I lay down. I let my pole in the water there and I lay down and I dozed off to sleep. And then all at once, I jumped up because somebody was there. I jumped up and I looked around and then I looked up. About halfway across, that little man was standing there, on that fallen tree. I thought maybe I was dreaming. I thought maybe it's not so. I really got up then. I wasn't asleep. And he said, "I'll be with you till the day you die." Those are the words he used. His toenails were long, but yet his hair was well kept. His hair was long but it wasn't dangling; it was real neat. And then he didn't have clothes but he had a kind of bandolier of plant leaves across in front. He stood up there, full-grown, his hair was neatly kept. The toenails are what I always remember. They were long; some of them were long and some of them were broken off. And he said, "I'll be with you till the day you die." That was my first encounter with him. I probably had to be around seven years old, because I was initiated at six and a half. It was after that. After that things started really happening. I was initiated, I was confirmed then into that category, and so they had already picked one for me, I guess.

I have seen him after that. Where I go and sit, my sacred ground, I have seen him, sitting right away from me a little ways, never said a word. I've seen him when I was looking for plants. I needed one right away and I didn't know just where to go. There was nothing said or spoken, but it seemed like he knew where I needed to go and I went. And then he said, "Over there, that's what you need." I remember him pointing at that, and he said, "Over there, that's what you need." I don't think I would normally have found it. He was actually showing me the plant that I was looking for. But it is not often, not often that I see him. I think they want you to see that they are still around so that you know that they are still around. The thing about it is they never change. I have never seen him grow any older. Still the same as the way I saw him the first time. And it was the same one I saw that night at my house.

NIGHT VISIT

My mistake was to mention the little people in a negative way. I guess it didn't go over too good with the little man himself. Chester Scott was at the church house when I went to visit my dad and he was working on the camp house that he was going to build for his mother. I usually took some extra boards that I had left over to give to him so that he could do his project. While we were there, he took a break and we were sitting around and we started talking about the little people. He was asking me questions about the little people. He told me he had heard a lot about them but he had never seen one. And I said, "Well, maybe they no longer exist, maybe they are not around anymore." That was the wrong thing to say.

When I got home and went to bed that night, in the middle of the night, somebody grabbed me by my hair and gave it a big yank and I woke up. I thought it was the kids' mother doing that and so I turned around and I looked over there but she was sound asleep and I knew that wasn't her. So I fixed my pillow there, I straightened up my pillow and then I made myself comfortable and I started to go back to sleep. Just as I settled down to go back to sleep, it really got a hold of my hair, I mean it really shook me then. This time I jumped up. I thought it was her, and I was going to catch her. But it wasn't her, she was asleep. She didn't even move. So I turned around.

On the window sill there, that little man I had seen many years ago was sitting down, his feet hanging down. There was anger in his voice. He said, "I'm real." And then he said it again, he said, "I'm real." Just like that. And then in a twinkle of an eye he was gone. So I knew better than to talk in a negative way because we try not to do that. They say they'll be with you. Those are your helpers. In time of need, hey, they'll come through. They'll show you plants. When you think you cannot find a plant, it is said that your helper, that means the little people, will actually show you what you are looking for. You will always find it because you will be shown.

That was a good experience because I wasn't sleeping, I sat straight up and, boy, he said, "I'm real. I'm real." You could tell he was angry from the voice. He was mad. I think I was trying to be nice to my friend who asked about the little people because he was saying he had never seen them, he had heard a lot about it. I think I was saying (I didn't say it right) it wasn't meant for him to see. Instead of wording it that way, I said maybe they weren't around anymore. I should have said, "It was never meant for you to see. You are not the right person for it. That is why you don't see." But instead I said maybe they weren't around anymore. And that was the night the little man let me know that he was real.

THANKING THEM

When my dad was dying, I sat up there and talked to him a few times. And when I came back the last time, he talked about the medicine. Did I remember all the things he had taught me? I said, "Yes. I know it all. I haven't forgotten anything. And I will carry it out like you taught me."

He said, "Use that medicine to help people with." I said, "That is the only way I know how, the way you taught me." And he got through saying that and he closed his eyes and took his last breath.

I thought about it way afterward. Why would he ask me if I knew my medicine? He knew that I was pretty good at that time. He knew that I knew the medicine, but he wasn't talking about the medicine to help people with. I think he was talking about the part that my grandmother and dad always said never to cry when an initiated person dies. And he was an initiated person. That was the part that he was actually asking. When I think back, I think he wasn't talking about medicine; he wanted to know if I knew that I was not supposed to cry. He knew he was dying. He just didn't come out and say it. That is what he was talking about. He wanted to make sure I knew everything he taught me, that I would also remember that part. That is what he was asking me.

I know that when my grandmother died, she was well-known and well liked, very popular. At the funeral, I guess everybody at the church house was crying. I guess I was the only one who didn't shed a tear. I have always remembered. After everybody had viewed the body, they closed the door and let the immediate family sit there a while. I have always remembered I whispered to her, "Just rest in peace. We'll meet again another day." I told her then, "It was very hard, but I did not shed a tear for you today. You taught me that. I learned well." That funeral, I heard a lot of rumors afterward. They said, "He must not even care about his Mama, he didn't even cry." They were talking about my grandmother. But they don't know I cried on the inside. I probably cried harder than any of them, but it was on the inside. The same thing happened with Dad. Everybody, my sisters, my family, everybody cried. I never did shed a tear for him. I did just like I did with my grandmother. I whispered to him. I said, "I passed your last test. You know what I am made of." Because that is what he was asking me that day. He wanted to know what I was made of when he was talking to me that day before he died. Would I hold up to what I was taught? And I reminded him. I said, "I passed your last test."

Afterward I went to the woods to the place that I always go to, the sacred ground. And I called both my grandmother and dad back, the last time together, and I thanked them for everything they had done for me. And I reminded them. I said, "I have gone through many tests and I have no problem with these tests, the four days' fast. I have been tested many times, but you two gave me the hardest test of all. And I think I did well. I hope I pleased you, both of you." And that is when my grandmother started rubbing her hand in my hair. My dad cleared his throat. So I know they were listening. That was the last test, after they were gone, that was the last thing they had thrown at me. I told them. "I carried out my end. I stood your test. You gave me the hardest test I would ever face. But you taught me well. I learned. I hope I pleased you." That was the final test that I went through. It was good. They wanted to see if I would cry because they said don't you ever do that; a main medicine man does not do that. Never cry for another initiated person. They had already gone through it. They knew how rough it was for them and now they were testing me. How I would do? Even deceased, they gave the final test to me.

No matter what you had done that was good, they never praised you for it. They never said, "You did real good." I have never heard that in my life, but when they were pleased, they looked at you and just smiled. That was all. That was all you needed to know. They never did say, "You did good. You did this and that." They just smiled and that was the unspoken word; they were pleased.

Chapter Six

THE STORY

This is the sacred story I was taught by my grandmother and my dad. It tells why we practice the medicine this way, the origins of the medicine plants, the pact between the medicine people and the plants, and the selection of the replacement for an initiated medicine person. We are forbidden to give the story away, but by leaving out parts of the story, the story will never all be told. It is all right to talk about two plants. The ceremonial ground uses red root all the time in the summer, but they don't know where it began to grow and how it came about. I want them to know how it got its name.

These things were given to us by the Creator; this is the consensus given by the more notable medicine people. Convictions such as these have their roots in a mystic past that predates history. There is no such premise or idea that the medicine people tried this or tried that until something worked. Knowledge of songs and herbs was either handed down or revealed by vision. All the plants have an origin, a beginning. For each of the plants that we use in our medicine world, the story tells how it began to grow, how it came about.

HOW THE MVSKOKE GOT THEIR MAIN MEDICINES

Long ago, there was a great Holy Man who lived some distance from a tribal town of our people. It is said that the people did not know where he came from, nor did they inquire. This Holy Man, they say, was very powerful for he could make people well by touching them with his hands.

It was the custom of the Mvskoke people to meet the needs of their holy men. They would bring food, till or care for his garden, repair or build his house. Whatever he needed to be done, it was the duty of the people to take care of the Holy Man. This was done out of love and great respect.

One day as he was passing through the village he noticed a young boy. The Holy Man had seen that this boy was mistreated and was kind of an outcast. He also knew that this boy was the kind of person that could learn the sacred ways that the Holy Man must pass on. So the Old Man took the boy to teach him the medicine ways and the sacred ways.

The Holy Man said: "I have seen the purity of your heart and know you will keep the sacred ways of healing and not misuse the power which

I have given you. For every healing chant shown to the chosen one, he is also shown a destructive word. There will be others selected just as I have selected you. The time is coming when you too will select a sole replacement to carry on the sacred way for your people."

The boy said: "Will the sole replacement be a boy or a girl?"

The Holy Man responded: "You know not if it is going to be a boy or girl, but the medicine people will know by a sign if the child can be selected."

The Young Man asked: "Why do I have to look for a sign to select my replacement?"

The Holy Man said: "So you will know the future of that child, what that person will be like until he dies. You will be shown what you need to use so the child will learn and not forget."

The boy made a comment: "With all the power that you have, will I have the same kind of power that enabled you to heal?"

The Holy Man said: "You will be able to do the things that are provided for you. In your dreams, you will be told the type of medicine and the chants and how to use them."

The boy had in his mind that he would have the power the Holy Man had. That is why the Holy Man had to keep telling him, bringing him back to nature. The boy was not going to have his power. He would need the help of the plants and animals.

The Holy Man just slowly turned to him and answered him: "Be patient. All things the chosen people will ever need to know to carry on after I'm gone have been laid out for all the medicine people to follow. The chosen people will have a choice of selecting their helpers (carriers), but the helpers will be limited to what the chosen ones will be willing to give and share with them. Carriers will not be given the origin of the medicine way, will not see new cures in visions but must maintain a strict disciplined way of life for the good of their people."

The Holy Man continued: "The medicine people will not have the power to heal by touch. Only I have been given that power. The medicine people will use what is shown in their dreams and visions and what has been put on this Mother Earth for them to use. All of their words will be built around three things which will always be here: human beings, animals, and plants. The sacred words are to have a sound of nature such as the sound of the wind or the cry of an animal."

And he said: "I have shown and taught you all the things you will need to help your people now and I will show you the new cures of the future in time. Be prepared to receive my instructions at all times, just as all medicine people must follow more instructions in the future."

The Holy Man noticed that the young man was curious why they always went to that certain place. The Holy Man said: "You have been wondering about this place for some time so I'll tell you why we meet here. This is a sacred ground and negative energies cannot come within the boundary of the four sacred poles in the ground. All selected medicine people will also have a sacred ground. All negative things are blocked out within that square. Within this square you will be able to communicate with me. This is where you will purify the sacred words and strengthen them. This is where you will strengthen your body and your mind in order to be prepared to receive any instruction which I might give at any time.

"There will be a time when medicine people will find their mate and this is where they will unite.[1] All the negative things will be left out. Within this square, there will be a circle, enough space for the two to step in and once both step in, they put their medicine down and close the circle. When they close the circle, everything they have done, good or bad, is locked in the circle. Everything else is locked out. Each has the power to remove the past from the other, just these two. Each one of them will have a feather. The woman will put one in the man's hair and she will remove all the things of yesterday. The man does the same thing. In case there's a time when this woman cannot bear a child for him to carry on, he would have the right to choose another mate, but once they have been in that circle, that woman will live with him the rest of their lives."

The Holy Man showed and taught him about the sacred ground. The young man was told to make one. So the Holy Man told the young man he was to go fast four days at his sacred ground and then come back to him and he would tell him more things. The boy told him: "I will get thirsty. I will get hungry. I will get sleepy." The Holy Man said: "All these sacred words that you keep holy will take care of you. When you are sleepy, the words are your sleep. Whenever you are hungry, that is your bread. Whenever you are thirsty, that is your water. This is why you keep these words sacred and they will take care of you in time of need."

The Holy Man said to the young man: "You know the purpose of a sacred ground. You purify the sacred word, strengthen your body and mind. Keep in mind, when problems arise and there seem to be no answers, come and communicate with me and get some of your answers to your problems. There is one more thing I must ask you to do. You must go and build a sweat house as near as possible to a running water. This will be a place only a chosen medicine person will be able to use. You will be shown the things that are to be used and the sacred words to use in preparing for sweat. In this sweat house you will expel impurity from within in form of a water. As you sit and sweat you must also sing the sacred song you have learned. As you sing, these sacred words will be washed and purified. When you have finished what you have been instructed to do, you will quickly go to the running water and wash off the impurity that has been expelled from within in form of a water. I asked you to build a sweat as near as possible to a running water for an important reason. You must never let the sweat on your body dry on you. The water will carry away all your impurity of your body."[2]

The time came when the Old Man said that he had to go away. And so, the time came when one last time they would sit and talk like they had done many times before. The Old Man recounted many things to the boy and what he must do. The Old Man was sitting where he always sat when he would tell the boy of good things, even funny things, but most of all, very serious sacred teachings. He said that if the boy was troubled at any time, he should remember that the Old Man would always be with him and to come back to where they sat and talked, and he would find the answer there and everything would be all right. This was very sad for the Old Man, but he was happy also for he had taught the boy and had someone to take his place.

Now it was necessary for him to leave, for his work was done. As their day together came to an end, the birds and the little things that make noises seemed to sound very lonesome. The Old Man bowed his head and began to cry and as he shed great tears, they fell to the ground and became a pool of tears. The Old Man held up his hand to the east and said: "This is the Blood of Life." The blood fell to the ground and made a small pool. His life was on the ground in tears and blood; only a great love and sadness would make this happen. Now he must leave. They said goodbye and the Holy Man left. The boy wanted to go with him so he ran after him, but could not find him. He tried to find his tracks but the Old Man left none. He disappeared.

Days went by and the boy helped the people with his powers and shared many sacred ways with them. One day the people became ill with a very bad illness. The boy tried to heal them by touching them with his hands. This did not work. The people became increasingly ill. The boy became very troubled and remembered what the Holy Man had told him, so he returned to the place where the Old Man had lived and to the place where they had sat when the Old Man went away. The old place was still familiar, recalling old times. The boy felt the Old Man was still there. But there was something different about the place where they had sat, for there were two bushes in front of the place where the Old Man had sat. The boy immediately knew that these plants were sacred medicines, for one bush grew from the place where his blood had fallen to the ground.

When placed in water, the roots of the bush that grew from the blood made the water red in color. Water remained clear or white when the roots of the bush that grew from the tears were placed in it. The boy knew that the Old Man was with him as he had said, for in his spirit he knew he was to use these sacred plants. He prepared himself and the medicines. He then took the medicines and cured the people of the great illness. To this very day these medicines remain sacred and are used by the Mvskoke people.

The name by which the Holy Man was called was because he was a great Holy Man and passed through the tribal towns of the people and lived a distance from them. His name was *Mēkko-hoyvnēcv* or "King passing through." The bush or the roots that grew from his blood is called by the same name today and is commonly known to the Mvskoke people as "red root."

The sacred bush and its roots that grew from the Holy Man's tears is called *Heles-hvtke* or "white medicine." This medicine is known to non-Indians as American ginseng.

THE STORY OF THE GATHERING

This young man had a dream. In this dream he was told that there would be a big gathering, that he would be surrounded by many, and he was told that he would be given instructions that he would follow. The dream did not mention whether the many would be men. The young man thought it would be people.

When he woke up the next morning, he thought it was a very strange dream that he had had. And he said: "Where will all these people come from? Where will the gathering take place and why are they going to gather?" Those are things that he was thinking about at that time. It bothered him for a little while, but then he forgot about it. It was just a dream.

The time came for him to do his annual fast and sweat. When he got to his sacred ground, there was something strange. It wasn't the way that he had always seen it. There was something that wasn't just right. He sensed that there was something strange about that day. He sat down and he was hearing all the little night creatures, the birds and the crickets. He was hearing these little night creatures during the day. That's why he said: "This is strange, very strange." Then he looked up and he saw the birds flying over, circling. That was unusual for some of the birds were too far from the water. And he thought about that a while. He said: "That's very strange, the birds circling and these little night creatures chirping and singing during the day."

Then it hit him. "This is the day that I had the dream about that there would be a gathering." Then he looked up to the sky and told the Creator: "Now I know that this is the day that the gathering is to take place. I am ready for the instructions and I will obey." When the sun was getting high, he was looking for people but he didn't see anybody. Then the sun was getting low and he was still thinking of people because he looked around and said: "Where are all these people? They should be getting here." He didn't know where they were to come from. Then he thought maybe he was wrong. Maybe it was not the day of the gathering. Then, the breeze in his face and the breeze that was coming through the trees, it was almost as if it were singing. There was almost a song in the wind, in the breeze. Then he said: "It's not people the dream was talking about." He said: "All of these things that are around me, the plants and all, these are the things the dream was telling me when it said that I would be surrounded by many." And then he repeated: "Whatever instruction is to be given out, I am ready."

All the medicine people that go to a sacred ground, they use medicine there and then they settle down. He had already used his medicine so he was ready for anything; he was ready for any instruction to be given and he would obey. Well, that's when he heard the voice. He was told: "You can move around, you are mobile. We are not." He knew the voice was the trees, the plants, whispering to him. "You can go to places a lot faster than we can. We are permanent. But in time, when you need us, you will also find us there. We'll also be there." (That is why the plants that were here before, next time you see the plants they're in another place. If you ever need them, the plants will begin to grow there too.) And there was a pact made then.

The whisper he heard said: "You have the power. You were given the power to heal with sacred words. We also have been given the power to heal. We are equal; we have the same power you have. The medicine people and the plants working together, we will be able to cure people. We will make a pact with you." The young man answered that he would accept the pact. The voice gave him the words to a chant. "These words you will use and we will listen to you. These words will be used before you remove us from this Mother Earth. You meet us halfway and we will meet you halfway. These are the sacred words you will say to us and when you use them, we will listen to what you say and then you have the power to remove us from this Mother Earth." With that permission, the plant was saying that we will meet you halfway and we will listen.

And the young man answered: "I will follow your instructions. I will use these sacred words before I ever remove you from this Mother Earth. I too will meet you halfway and we will work together to cure our people."

And so the plants answered back and said: "From this day on, all the medicine people will be known as the keepers of the plants."

So this is how it is going to be. All the medicine people will be keepers of the plants. The actual words of the chant that they use before removing plants were given to that man. Most of the time medicine people are shown what to do through vision, but this time the plants said this. This is the only time a plant gave instructions to a human being.

It started when that Holy Man made a selection. He taught the boy about the plants. He was really prophesying about a lot of things. The prophecy was that the plants were going to be used: You will be shown what plants to use in your visions. You will watch the tree from seedling to maturity and then it will get old and die right before your eyes. You will also be shown the sickness, the symptoms of particular sicknesses. These will be the plants that you will use. Then you will be given the sacred words to use for each sickness. In other words, you will be shown the plants, the symptoms, and the chants at the last.

In books, it always says this was learned by trial and error. There was no trial and error for the old people. They already knew exactly what they were going to use.[3]

THE STORY OF THE BIRDS

Now the young man had made a pact with the plants, and he was well satisfied, but he thought about this for a long time. He thought about the voices that he had heard. He said: "They are alive just as I am. They too get tired, just like I get tired. I was given the responsibility to take care of these plants. They too will need a rest. How do I give these plants a rest?" He thought about it a long time and he remembered the birds in the sky. "All animals that fly, that have wings, will be the carriers. They will have the chore of bringing the changing weather."

So he called them all together. They were gathered, and he gave them a choice. He didn't say certain ones would migrate south; they had the choice. "You will bring in the changing of weather in order that these plants may rest. As you begin to migrate south you will sing and let the trees and other plants throughout the land know that you are bringing a change of weather and to be prepared." Then the plants' leaves begin to fall. (So that's why when you hear these geese, these birds go by, they sing. They sing as they go to let the plants know that they are bringing in the changing weather.) The birds bring in the cold weather so that the trees will go dormant, giving the plants a chance to rest. All the sap, life-sustaining minerals and substances that they have inside them will have a chance to go back to the ground, to Mother Nature, to purify itself again and come back again come spring. Just like the medicine men who always clean themselves to keep strong, the plants are no different. The young man told the birds: "You will sing as you come back and the plants will hear you. They will awaken."

The migrating birds will be responsible for bringing in the cold, and they will bring back the warmth for the plants to grow again when it is time. (You notice that it is almost four months, November, December, January, and February, that the plants are dormant.)

Then, he went a little further. He told the birds that didn't leave that they were being given a choice again, which birds will stay up at night. "I need the birds of the night to watch over the people throughout the night. You will be up all night." Then he gave the other birds the chore of being the ones to relieve these birds of the night. They would rise early in order that the others can rest and they will take over from there the rest of that day. That is why they are already up before the sun's up; the birds are already doing their work. So the birds are up twenty-four hours. You've got some during the day, then the night birds take over.

Everything that we do is built around plants and animals. Everything that we do, the medicine way, it's all built around Mother Nature.

Chapter Seven

PLANTS

These are some of the plants used by my family and also mentioned in John Swanton's Religious Beliefs and Medical Practices of the Creek Indians. The final four are not names of plants, but they are in Swanton's plant list. Swanton does not mention any comments by my great grandfather, Jackson Lewis, for these last four (see also appendix B).

1. Mēkko-hoyvnēcv

King passing through, red root   *Salix humilis*

Mēkko-hoyvnēcv translates in Mvskoke as "King passing through." In English the Mvskoke call it red root since the roots soaked in water turn the water red. We go out and locate what we want and we get it out of the ground and if possible, if there is a running stream there we try to wash them off while we are still out in the woods, and then we cut it to the length that we want, that we are going to store. We bring it home and then we use a hammer just to pound it, to knock the bark off; we lay the bark out and let it dry itself naturally before we ever put them up. Some of those things require you to prepare them without eating, and some you have to use within four days after they come out of the ground. It is no good if you don't. Those we don't store. We use them right away. I go out and pick some early in the morning and I'll come back and I'll strip it down right there and then fix the medicine. But the rest of the roots you can store. *Mēkko-hoyvnēcv* is used for many sicknesses and can be used internally, externally, hot or cold. The songs will be different. The medicine is made the same way if used hot or cold or internally or externally. If used hot, the patient takes it home and heats it.

Uses:

(a) It is used for doctoring the houses. Enough is made to sprinkle the house out four times completely. The medicine person puts the roots in a jar, adds water, and sings the right chants facing east, using the medicine stick. The medicine is used cold to remove all negative things out of the house. Sprinkling the house itself could be done either by the person asking for it or the medicine person could be called to their home to do it.

(b) *Mēkko-hoyvnēcv* is used to clean a person out if it is believed something has been done, the person has been witched. You give such people the medicine to drink while they are standing in a running water such as a stream and let them vomit into the water, cleansing them out.

(c) It is used on a person that has mental stress or is worried to a point of being out of harmony with nature. He or she washes with the medicine (hot or cold, depending on which chants you use). To wash with it, the person is instructed to wet their head, face, and back of their neck and let it dry naturally. This must be done for four days in a row.

(d) This is one of the main medicines at the ceremonial ground for cleansing. Participants drink it and vomit.

2. Passv

Button snake root, bear grass   *Eryngium yuccifolium*

To make *passv*, gather the whole plant, roots and top, and put it in water and sing the chants with the medicine stick. Which chants are used depends on if the medicine is to be used hot or cold, who is using it, and what the ailment is.

Uses:

(a) The Mvskoke use it during the Green Corn Dance. The medicine man prepares the medicine and the participants, using their first two fingers, dip their fingers into the medicine, make an offer to the four directions, and drink some of the medicine.

(b) It is used in a different way at the beginning of the Green Corn Ceremony to prepare for the ceremony. The medicine man dips a needle or thorn or anything sharp like that in the medicine and then he scratches the person. After the person is scratched, the medicine man takes a branch and slaps the scratched arm, leg, back, or whatever part was scratched.

(c) *Passv* is used on children to expel worms. They drink a prepared medicine that induces vomiting or the passing through of a natural bowel movement.

(d) It can be used for treating venereal disease, for which people drink the medicine and wash the affected area.

(e) It is used also for treating rheumatism by warming the medicine and applying it to the affected area with a cloth dipped and wrung out.

(f) *Passv* is used very effectively on a person who has high fever. Drinking the medicine and getting by a hot fire until he or she sweats takes the fever out.

3. Heles-hvtke

White medicine   *Ginseng*
        Panax quinquefolium

Uses:

(a) This is used for shortness of breath by boiling the roots and giving the liquid to patients and letting them vomit.

(b) It is used in conjunction with soap for a body wash to remove a bad spell done to a person. Prepare it by cutting up the soap into your water. Scrape the roots of *heles-hvtke* real fine and put the scrapings (a powder) in water and sing the chant. Then the person washes the hair and body. It is used for four consecutive days.

(c) *Heles-hvtke* is used in making a medicine bag for good luck or protection. You always put red roots with this in something good. You scrape the root and get a fine powder and put a little in with all medicines that are for good purposes. It represents purity. We use it for good things to happen.

(d) It is used after a heart attack. The medicine person uses the whole root in water, usually in a quart jar, and chants. The sick person takes a small drink once a day or any time if not feeling right, adding water until the root disintegrates, then getting more from the medicine man. A person who has had a heart attack will always need that medicine for the rest of his or her life. Science has not found anything beneficial in this, but we use it. People in the Orient use it. It is not only the medicine but the chants that make it work. We use it for heart attack. This is a basic medicine for the Mvskoke. I have not seen anyone die of heart attack who uses this.

4. Notossv

Purplestem Angelica   *Angelica atropurpurea*

We use strictly the roots. They are very bitter roots and those can be stored. In fact I've still got some that Dad had. All these medicines made with *notossv* are made with the roots only. Now we also have chants, different chants, with all of these.

Uses:

(a) This is used on children to expel worms. You put the root in the water, soak it in water. It is very bitter; you don't let it get too bitter and you let them drink that. Or they can chew it and swallow the juice of it, but it is bitter if you do it that way, real bitter. So it is better to put it in water.

(b) It is used on adults to cure back pain. Put the root in water and make them drink that.

(c) *Notossv* is used by women during the Green Corn Ceremony Ribbon Dance to prevent heat stroke. You soak the root in water and they take a sip of that.

(d) The ceremonial singers during the Mvskoke ceremonies and the drummers during the pow-wow ceremonies in other tribes use this. They chew the root. The medicine person prepares the root by holding it, turning it around in his hand as he sings and spits on it. He does not use a medicine stick.

(e) You can use it for relieving stomach disorder by chewing the root and swallowing the juice.

(f) We use it to get someone off or to prevent a person from going to jail. It is also used against lawsuits. The medicine person scrapes the roots real fine and sprinkles on tobacco with *heles-hvtke*. Then you open up a package of cigarettes, hold them in your hand, and turn them over. Sprinkle the medicine on the end of the cigarettes that will burn. Or, if using a bag of pipe tobacco, sprinkle the medicine into the bag.

The medicine person talks to the clients. Say they are charged with something but they are going to deny it. The medicine man needs to know if they did it. You talk to them and find out if the charge is true or not. The reason you have to know is there is a difference in the chant that may be used to make the medicine. There is a chant to use if the client is telling the truth and wants them to believe him. There is a different chant if the person is lying but wants them to believe he is telling the truth.

The client smokes at least one cigarette a day for four days. He can then smoke the rest at any time but he saves one or two to be smoked on the court date. He is to brush his clothes down with smoke and get it all over himself. He can smoke the last one outside the court building but needs to smoke the last one on the court day. He does not have to smoke two that day. I get more demands from non-Indians for this than from Indians.

5. *Welanv*

Wormseed   *Chenopodium ambrosioides*

In Swanton's book, *Religious Beliefs and Medical Practices of the Creek Indians*, Jackson Lewis wouldn't make a statement on this one. I wonder why because this is one of our most basic medicines. That tells me that he wasn't all that enthused about giving information to anyone.

Uses:

(a) This plant is used for purifying the ceremonial ground during the Green Corn thanksgiving dance. Sprigs are used to sweep under each arbor.

(b) It is very effective for getting rid of intestinal worms in young children. The whole plant (leaves, stems, and roots) is boiled and given to the child to drink. The child is to drink only a small amount of the liquid.

(c) In an older person, it is used for relieving very high fever. The leaves and stems of this medicine are boiled and the liquid is given to people while still warm, making them sweat to relieve the fever. They drink this, but you could also pour it on them. You have them standing outside, facing east, and you pour it on them. It will get the high fever out of them that way too. My grandma used that quite a bit, having them stand out there and then pouring it on them, and it sure got the fever out of them.

(d) *Welanv* is good for sore eyes. The roots are gathered from the east side of the plant. Enough is gathered to be used for four days. You put the root in water and sing using the medicine stick. Then the eyes will be washed out with the medicine. The chant used depends on if the medicine is to be used hot or cold. There are four different chants. One is for medicine to be used warm for eyes that are sore and red, and a second one is for medicine to be used cold for eyes sore and red. There is a third chant for medicine to be used warm if the eyes burn and things look foggy, and a fourth for medicine to be used cold if the eyes burn and things look foggy.

6. Vcenv

Cedar   *Juniperus sp.*

This is one of the main medicines for the Mvskoke people. A beautiful story is told by the main medicine people of the origin of this tree.

Uses:

(a) We use the sprigs in conjunction with many other plants for many different kinds of sickness, in medicines to be used hot or cold.

(b) *Vcenv* is used to treat pain and aches or swelling of the joints. The sprigs and leaves are heated together in water, and the water and the sprigs and leaves are applied warm.

(c) It is used for purification of homes by smoking the house out. It is used in conjunction with tobacco. You get wood chips to burning to make a coal and sprinkle the cedar sprigs and leaves, tobacco, and *heles-hvtke* on the wood chips to induce smoke. Then smoke the yard and house for purification, to get rid of unwanted things.

7. Kvpvpaskv

Spicewood, spicebush   *Lindera benzoin*

Uses:

(a) If red roots are scarce, this plant is one of the main substitutes used for cleansing for people who have been to a funeral and also for the one who dug the grave. It is used cold. Usually they just put it on the porch or whatever and when people come by, they wash with it. You use the leaves or the whole top of the plant. You squash it all up and put it in water.

(b) The leaves can be put in water and used to take a bath by people who are worried, causing stress. This medicine can be used hot or cold. It depends on the season. In wintertime you want them to use it hot. Lots of times they'll ask for it hot, regardless of the season. You use different chants for hot and for cold.

8. Kofockv-rakko

Horsemint *Monarda sp.*

These medicines are used in liquid form and you use the top part of the plant. We usually just cut it up and put it all in water all together. We don't use the roots. It is made cold, but the chants are for hot or cold. If it is for hot, they take it home and boil it, or heat it up.

Uses:

(a) We use this for back pain by warming the medicine and applying to the sore spot for four days.

(b) It is used for joint pain by applying medicine to the sore spot. This can be used hot or cold. The chants are different.

(c) Tribal ground shell shakers use this medicine for swelling of the feet and legs by washing and soaking their feet in the medicine. It can be used hot or cold, depending on the chant.

(d) *Kofockv-rakko* can be used to cure mental stress by washing and taking a bath in the medicine. The person uses it for four days.

(e) This plant is used a lot in conjunction with *heles-hvtke* for doctoring a house or cleansing around it. This is done by sprinkling all the rooms of the house.

(f) We use this on people who tend to sleep a lot. There are people who want to sleep all the time. You have them wash with it and drink a small amount. They use it cold.

9. Kvtohwv

Honey locust *Gleditsia triacanthos*

Uses:

(a) We use the bark in conjunction with *mēkko-hoyvnēcv* and *heles-hvtke*; this is used for good luck by the Mvskoke. It is put into a medicine bag, sewn, or tied in a leather pouch.

(b) The bark is used in conjunction with *mēkko-hoyvnēcv* to treat varicose veins. You put the bark in water. You pour the medicine on the legs and rub downward away from the body.

(c) The roots can be used to stupefy fish. You pound the roots and throw them into the water.

10. Vlv

Buckeye *Aesculus sp.*

Uses:

(a) *Vlv* is used for people who have cataract problems. You do this by getting on the top side of the limb. Scrape the top part of the limb and put it in water. Normally, you dip a finger in that medicine and get

the water of the medicine in your eye. It is kind of like washing the eyeball
with it but with a very small amount.

(b) The seed from the buckeye is for good luck. First you purify the
seed. You get your water in a little jar and put red roots in it. Use a little,
short medicine stick and sing the chant and blow into the jar. This is the
medicine for purifying the *vlv*. Dip two fingers in the medicine and sprinkle
a seed that you are holding in your hand as you turn the seed over. Sprinkle
it four times. So the seed is purified. There are chants for good luck and
for protection. Facing east, hold the seed in your hand and roll it over at
all times as you sing the chants. At the end of each chant, you spit on the
seed. Each chant is sung four times. Sew the seed into a little bag to wear
around the neck or carry it in a purse or pocket.

11. Haloneske or aloneske
Devil's shoestring   *Tephrosia virginiana*
Uses:
(a) The roots are used same as *kvtohwv* or honey locust to treat varicose veins.

(b) The plant is also used in shallow creeks to stupefy fish. The roots
are pounded up and put into water.

(c) This is very effective for treating a person who has been shot with
a gun. You pound the plant roots into fine powder and put them in water
and warm the water and wash the affected area.

12. Vtakrv-lvste
Black weed   *Baptisia sp.*
Use:
Fresh roots are used to treat a person that has diarrhea. Some of them
will lose a lot of weight real fast, dehydrating. Put the roots in water and
give them about half a cup to drink three to four times a day until it stops.
This is used cold.

13. Cvto-heleswv
Rock medicine
The client will have an actual rock that you work on for the first two uses.
It is not a plant. They get it out of running water, a real smooth rock, and
they usually get it themselves and bring it. We use different things like the
cedar; we smoke the rock down and the chants are done. Then we give it
back to them and they carry it in their pocket.
Uses:
(a) This medicine is used when a person wants to be noticed by other

people and to stand out.

(b) The person who has a heavy thought about things that need to be done which are good will use this medicine to get other people to give him support.

Now there is also a plant called *Cvto-heleswv*, rock medicine. You use the leaf part; put it in the water and people use it to rinse the mouth out for sore tonsils. They don't drink it; they just gargle.

14. *Yvnvsv-heleswv*

Bison medicine

Uses:

(a) A man will take a bath with this medicine when he is going to play a stickball game. They would use it before playing the east and west game or playing against another tribe or against another tribal ground. The medicine is made of the leaves and roots. You put them in water. Normally it is used cold.

(b) Small kids are given a bath with this medicine to make them strong and husky as they grow. You are using the same parts of the plant that you use for the medicine in the stickball game, but the chant is different. The stickball game medicine is getting them prepared to play stickball. In other words they will take a beating and yet at the same time they have got to hold up, not fatigue out. For the small kids, you are giving them a bath so they will be strong and husky. So it is two different chants for the two different medicines, yet the plant does the same thing.

15. 'To-heleko

Mistletoe   *Phoradendron sp.*

For all of these you use the top, the leaves. It is a parasite anyway. There is no root.

Uses:

(a) This is used to clear passages to the lungs for easier breathing. It is used in conjunction with *mēkko-hoyvnēcv*. They are boiled and the sick person covers the head with a towel to inhale the vapor of the medicine.

(b)For this one, the leaves are put into water by the medicine person during the night. The medicine has to be made without the medicine person eating that day, so you prepare it after midnight. You don't eat from midnight until you make the medicine. It is for a person who complains of having trouble sleeping.

(c) It is used for treating hemorrhoids by boiling the leaves and using a "star shit" (*kolaswv-holvnwv*) like a little sponge. Soak the *kolaswv-holvnwv* in the medicine and apply to the rectum. You put 'to-heleko in the water and say the chants and they take it home and boil it and then dip the *kolaswv-holvnwv* in the liquid and apply it.

(d) Women are given this for their cramps during the monthly period. This is not recommended for carriers to use on women unless they are thoroughly knowledgeable about how to administer it. The main problem is you could give it to people and it is way too bitter. Instead of helping them, you hurt them. The more you boil it, the more bitter it gets. It is delicate to get it just right. The woman drinks it. It has to be just right because if it is too strong, she will have a different reaction to it because a lot of juice comes out of the leaves. That is why you don't let carriers do this because they have to have been using this medicine over and over again to know exactly what it is like. You can tell by the color of it, but they don't know that. You let the person drink a little of that. It doesn't take much.

(e) People that have been bedridden for a long time are given baths four times a day with this. For this it is used cold.

(f) People who pass blood when they urinate are given a small dose of this medicine to drink. It can be used warm (not hot) or cold.

(g) It is called "the little people's medicine." The reason it is called this is that the little people use this medicine to keep themselves strong and clean in order to help the medicine person that they have selected to help until that medicine person dies.

16. Akhatkv

White down in (the bottom)   *Sycamore*

Platanus occidentalis

You use the bark and put it in water for all of these.

Uses:

(a) *Akhatkv* is used for the fast healing of broken bones. It is applied to the broken bones by pouring on or soaking the affected area. It can be used hot or cold.

(b) Also some parents will use this medicine to make a child light complected by giving them a bath with this medicine.

(c) It is good for eyes when the eyeballs start to get white spots. You wash with it like with the cataract medicine.

17. Akcelvlaskv

White birch   *Betula sp.*

For both of these medicines you use the bark and put it in water.

Uses:

(a) *Akcelvlaskv* and *Akwahnv* (number 18) are used on people who are troubled or lonesome and for people who have lost their loved ones. The person is instructed to take a bath with this medicine just before bedtime for at least ten days. It can be used hot or cold.

(b) There is a medicine made with this that is used on people who are said to have spirits riding on their backs. It's a bad energy on their backs. This medicine is used warm and is poured on the person's back as they are standing facing east.

18. Akwahnv

Willow *Salx sp.*

Uses:

(a) This is used the same as described in the first cure for *Akcelvlaskv* (number 17a).

(b) If the *mēkko-hoyvnēcv* (red root) is not available, this is used as a substitute for vomiting or cleansing the person out.

19. Coskv

Post oak *Quercus stellata*

Use:

This is very effective for getting rid of sores on the legs and body. It is used in conjunction with *mēkko-hoyvnēcv*(red root). The bark of this tree and the roots of *mēkko-hoyvnēcv* are boiled and the person is given instructions to take a bath with this medicine for about fourteen days. This is for external use only.

20. Pvkanvho

Wild plum *Prunus sp.*

Uses:

(a) We use this for people who have sores on their face. The leaves are boiled and the person drinks the liquid.

(b) It is very effective for getting rid of spider bites or small bug bites. You wash the affected area with the medicine made by boiling the leaves.

(c) *Pvkanvho* is good for a person who has mumps, to reduce the swelling. The medicine person puts leaves in water. Heat it and use it on the affected area by applying a soaked cloth to the swelling.

21. Tvfosho

Elm *Ulmus sp.*

Uses:

(a) This is good for toothache. The inner bark is used but not the branches. The inner bark is put in water and the person seeking help will rinse the mouth out and take some of the inner bark and chew on it.

(b) For broken bones, you boil the inner bark and apply the liquid to a broken bone and it will heal fast. It can be used hot or cold.

(c) The inner bark is gathered from the east side of the tree and used to help a person with having bowel movements. This medicine is made by putting inner bark into a quart jar of water in conjunction with four small strips of *mēkko-hoyvnēcv* (red root). The chants are sung and blown through the medicine stick. Usually this is used cold. The person drinks this.

22. Pvrko-rakko

Big grape, summer grape   *Vitis palmata*
Use:
This is very effective when used on a person who tends to go out on their spouse. The tips of the vine, the part that clings to a tree or limbs, are taken and wrapped together with the hair of the person or spouse who is stepping out. This is buried in the front yard. The chant is very long for this medicine.

23. Tartahkv

Cottonwood   *Populus deltoides*
Use:
This medicine is known to heal broken bones fast in humans as well as animals such as mules or cows. Farmers use this a lot on animals. This can be used cold or hot, depending on the season. Soak the bark and pour the liquid on the broken area.

24. Wēso

Sassafras   *Sassafras sp.*
Uses:
(a) Sassafras is used for thinning blood. The roots are gathered from the east side of a tree and boiled to a color of tea and strained. A person is to take a cupful of this medicine in the morning and just before going to bed.

(b) It is given to a person with kidney problems to flush out the system. It is prepared the same as when used for thinning blood except the chant is different.

(c) Also it can be used for high blood pressure. It is made the same way as made for thinning blood, but red root is used with it and the chant is different.

25. Hece-pakpvke

Tobacco bloom   *Lobelia sp.*
Uses:
(a) This is used to doctor a ceremonial ground fire. You pour the

tobacco on the fire. The chants are said over the tobacco. I would use the tobacco dry but they had a lot of versions for different grounds, the way that it was used back then. In fact, that is probably one of the oldest; it is older than tobacco, really. But you don't see this plant anymore. The plants are very hard to locate. I haven't seen any in Oklahoma. I think they are gone in a way, in our area anyway. There might still be some in Alabama.

(b) The camps on the ceremonial ground are protected from bad spirits or negative things that could be inflicted on them. You could use the tobacco wet or dry. In a dry form, you have to blow on it with the chant. Or you could put it in a bucket with water. Either way you sprinkle it around.

26. Poyvfekcv-heleswv

Spirit medicine

There is no scientific name for this because this is not a plant. It is a problem that can be doctored. If people are talking about spirits bothering them, there is a medicine that we use for that. We make a medicine to correct a problem with the spirits. It is not a plant, but you use a plant; that is confusing right there. Suppose somebody is sleeping and hears somebody else come in. Or a person might say, "While I was lying there, somebody shook my leg or hand or pulled the cover off me." There is medicine for that and there are plants we use for that. But poyvfekcv-heleswv is not a plant.

27. Pesē-heleswv

Woman's breast medicine

This also is not a plant. It identifies systems or a problem that is to be doctored.

28. Efolo-heleswv

Screech owl medicine

This is not a plant. People are really afraid of any owl and there is medicine for the owl, to keep them away. The owl will come and alight on a tree right by their yard, and they will ask you for medicine to keep owls away. They will say, "We don't want them to come around."

29. Awvnhē-heleswv

The name *awvnhē-heleswv* means constipation, again not a plant.

Chapter Eight

MAKING MEDICINE

People take the medicine for granted now. I don't think they even have a lot of respect for medicine people. The only time that they really up and holler is when they've got to call in medicine people because they can't get any help on the outside from regular clinics and medical doctors. Whenever people say that their doctors give up on them and they know they can't get any help, then they really look for the medicine man. Then they really start searching. But that's the only time that they want to search and find somebody who can help. But the young ones nowadays, there isn't anybody here to teach them.

People say, "I wish I was one, a medicine man." They think it's real easy. They don't have any idea; it's a rough road. It's hard, with a lot of temptations. You've got to go out and do things that most people wouldn't do, especially in the wintertime. You wouldn't get just anybody to go out there and look for roots. When there's sleet and rain, nobody's going to leave the house, but there are times that you've got to because there's some roots you have to use freshly picked from the ground. And then you have to do it. It's not easy. But, you know, one thing about it: you don't ever get sick. You never catch a cold. You get wet and you don't even get sick from that. So, we must be doing something right. Somebody's taking care of us, too. It's pretty tiresome sometimes, though. You have to keep going and going and going all the time.

KEEPING STRONG

The first thing for a medicine person is that we keep ourselves strong. In order for our medicine to be strong, we have to be strong personally. That's the basic thing. In the story of the boy and the sweat, the Old Man told the boy that he had to be strong and his mind and body had to be clean. The story doesn't say clear, it says clean. And then when the boy asked, "How do I keep myself clean?" what he was talking about was how do I keep my mind clean? Actually, you do that by thinking in a positive way, not a negative way, everything positive. We do take our medicine regularly to keep ourselves strong. We do sweat. And that is to keep ourselves physically and mentally clean and strong. But at the same time that we do the sweat, we are also cleansing our chants, to keep them pure and clean. Keep them strong. We do fast once a year, four days. You could call it an endurance test because of what we're going through. We're getting ready to find out just how well we have taken care of all of these and in turn it, the medicine, will take care of us so that we can go through this with no problem. So it is more or less like a test at the same time.

When I go into the woods, I go into my sacred square and when I am in it I use my medicine and then I lean back and close my eyes. I can feel the energy change. I start to hear voices. I hear my grandmother's voice. I feel her combing my hair back with her fingers like she used to do when I was little. I also hear Dad's voice. I hear other voices too I can't identify. Some of them I think I know. They were in those last eight powerful medicine people. Others I don't know. If I open my eyes I can see objects. It looks foggy but I can make out a shape and just enough to recognize the person. They are all medicine people. Only medicine people can come in the square. They are encouraging me never to be weak. I can communicate with them if I choose to do so. I talk to my grandmother most of the time. I thank them for their support. I sit back and watch my whole life happen again before my eyes. It is just like I am sitting on a log looking down on it. I see myself being born, I hear them talk about me, and I see my grandmother and my dad teaching me. I go through the whole training process and see my initiations and getting my medicine sticks. I hear all the words. I watch my whole life right up to the present. This is one of the reasons we never forget. We can relive it every year just like it was happening yesterday. Most wonderful thing about this is that I can relive or bring back any year of my life for a little while.

On the third day I usually go to sweat and wash the words. Dad used to go on the fourth day. I go on third day. There is not a set time to go but you have to do it during the four days. You have to wash the words. Then the sacred fire and sacred water wash the words. You say them and they are washed. You have a choice of what words you may want to clean and as you sing, the words coming out of your mouth are being washed clean.

All of this process cleans your mind and your body, the time in the sacred square, the time in the sweat. You thank the medicine people for supporting you and helping you stay strong. And then you are tested; there is always a test of some kind within the four days and then it is sad when you have to leave and there you are alone again. Then I have to come back into your reality, this reality.

But after all of these fasts are over and you are getting back to your normal routine, that is when you are the strongest. You can tell what a person is going to say to you before they say it. In other words if they come for the medicine, you already know the problem or what they are going to ask you. Your mind is so fresh and strong, you're thinking that you actually know what that person is going to say to you before it ever happens. But you still listen to them.

Now Dad would beat them to it sometimes. Dad would tell them what they needed before they would tell him. He would tell them, "This is what you need; this is what you came after." I don't do that though. Dad did it. He did it often. But when we can do that, it tells us that we know we have kept ourselves strong in all ways, the way we are supposed to keep ourselves.

RELATIONSHIP WITH THE ANIMALS

One time I was coming back from Arkansas, stopping by Sallisaw in that park. I was tired. I leaned back against the tree and the women were over there at the table. I leaned back and I was going to sleep a little bit and then was going on home. There were some birds in the tree and I called one. It pecked around on the top of my head. One lit on my head there and I was just about to go to sleep and he slipped and his wing flapped me in the ear and I shook my head and scared him off. I called him back again. This time he stayed up there but every once in a while I could feel him sliding down. Then he would crawl back up there. He would pull my hair. When I woke up, he flew off.

Those women came over and said, "Did you know there was a bird in your hair?" I said, "Sure, I called him." That scared them and they jumped in the car and they left right then and there. But we can control some things. Animals, we can talk with them, we can handle them. It's no big deal though. See, to others it really means something. To me it would mean nothing. You don't see us go out and kill anything that it is not necessary to kill either. We take care of them; they take care of us. It works two ways. They probably thought I was a nut, those women, thought there's something wrong with this guy.

TESTING A MEDICINE PERSON

Those plants are very, very strange. Some of the people that call themselves medicine men have asked me to help them get certain roots. I have taken them out in the woods and taken them right up to the roots, the kind of plants that they're looking for, where they are plentiful out there. I have taken some of them right up to the plants so that they're standing right up against them. And then I would ask them, "There used to be plenty of them right here—do you see any?" And they would look and they'd say, "No, I guess they've picked them all. I don't see anything." And they'd be standing right up against that plant. When that happens, well, we have an old saying: "It was not meant for them to use it." They could not see that plant. They were standing right up against it.

But when that happens, we always say, "Well, they must've picked them all. They're just not here." I'll always take them away from there and say, "We'll go look somewhere else." But I never show them. I'll always tell them, "There used to be some right here." Because if it was meant for them to use it, they would have seen it. We know that. That's one of the ways that we have of testing people that say they are medicine people. We have many ways of testing people. There's no way they can beat us to that. There's no school on that. And we know who's who. We *have* to know.

DIAGNOSIS

We really don't have names like the medical terms that they have now. The Indians don't have medical terms for sickness. We go by how the person is affected, their symptoms, and we know what to use.

Most of the time medicine people will listen to a patient. We already have an idea of what we're going to do. I already know what people will probably need, but we do let them talk about all their symptoms. And then we will ask them what kind of medicine did the medical doctors prescribe to them, and what are the medical doctors going to do, and what are they being treated for? That's the main thing. That's one of the things we'll always ask. "What are they treating you for?" From what they're telling us, we're analyzing the way that it will affect people. We'll sit there and listen to, "The medical doctor says I need this because of this and that," and then we ask, "How do you actually feel? Where does it hurt? How often? How does it affect your body?" That's the thing we're getting at. We're listening to all of this, and that's where experience comes in because we've dealt with some of these. We're looking for the key thing that may change the whole thing around. But when they get through telling you all of these things here, then we say, "The thing that the medical doctors are giving you, your treatment (we don't ever tell them it's not going to help them—it's doing them some good up to a certain point), I would treat this in a different way. This is what I think is wrong. From what you just described to me, this is how your body's acting, this is what we use in order to get people well. This is a little different from what the medical doctors have said. I'm going to give you medicine that is different from what they've said."

We know what plants to use and which chants to use to go directly to a problem. These days the pharmacies have pills. Basically, the pills are the plants that we've been using for all these years. They just gave a medical word to them. That's all. That's the only difference. We use plants in the same way, barks, roots, and leaves. But now they've got it in tablets and they've got words for them. They've got medical terms for them. We don't have that. But they try to duplicate our stuff. It would be just like the sassafras we use; they can analyze everything, they can test those things and tell you exactly what's in them, and they can go out and follow it and make it in a synthetic way, until it's almost the same. But there's one thing I always tell those medical people. I say, "You know, you can always duplicate what we've got, but there's one thing we'll have only. You don't have chants to direct cures. We do. We know where we're going with ours. You don't. You've got to go by trial and error with yours. We don't have to do that."

A TREATMENT FOR SORES

For example, the relatives described to me what was wrong with a man. They were talking about sores all over his body, spreading. The medical doctor had been telling him, "We think this is what's wrong and so we're giving you this and this and that." Just types of medicine, but it wasn't working. Instead of getting better, he kept getting worse. So they called me and asked if I would look at him and see what could be done. From what I saw, I already had my idea of what I was going to make because of the way the sores were coming out. It was his blood system; the impurity in his body was so great that the wastes that are supposed to be removed from the body were not being removed by his kidneys, his liver, and bladder. Everything in there was not carrying out its work, moving out the impurity in his body. It had already had the body off balance, and his body couldn't take care of the wastes of the body fast enough so that it was mounting up, causing all that. So I used a simple thing. I won't mention the roots. There were two different roots I used. I made the medicine. I used the sassafras to kill the bitterness out of the other type of root. But that was to get it into his system to help the other vital parts of his body, to help it function to remove all of these impurities out of his body. And the medicine that I gave him was to clean his body out, remove it right away. And the response was in three days. It already started clearing up. That came about just from experience, I knew exactly what to give him. So I gave him something that his body would absorb into his system fast, and then help the body repair itself.

We removed all the impurity out of his body, so that his own system could pick that up. In other words, the body didn't have to work as hard. The man is getting old; the body doesn't work as good. So with the medicine, all the system was flushed out clean. And then his body could take over from there. It should be able to handle the rest of what it's supposed to do.

WEIGHT LOSS

Another example is a little girl thirteen years old who was losing weight. This was in Nebraska. They gave up on her, I guess, all the kinds of medical doctors down there in Nebraska and Colorado, but it was very simple. When her family came down and they talked to me and explained it, I said, "This is very simple. There's nothing to it." And then we just do what we're supposed to do. That little girl is going to school full time now, when before they said they didn't even want to fool with her at school. I talked to her. They called me. They said, "She hasn't missed her school. She's gained weight and she's in school." Those are things that medicine people don't talk about. They just go out and do it. That's why we listen to the people when something is wrong with them. We sit around, we listen. And they say, "We went to a medical doctor; this is what he told us." They'll give you the whole thing. But all the time you listen to what they're saying. Then when they get through you say, "This is the way I would do it, and this is what you want." Then you just go out and make medicine for them.

HEADACHE

If I were making something for headache, for example, I would probably use two different chants. We don't ever put more than two songs to any medicine. I've heard other people do three, four, but my family never used it. They always said just two was enough. Now if a woman was talking about headache, I would have a chant just for that particular thing, and then I would probably add one that would relax her at the same time. In other words, there are different songs for that, to ease her mind. It could be stress and so that is the thing that you have to analyze as they talk to you. What extra might you want to put in? And I would more likely think there is a lot of stress here. And so you would add one in there to ease her mind. So what you have done is you use two different chants.

If she asked for it hot, then you do the headache medicine using the words that are supposed to be used for hot. If she asked for something that she wants to use cold, there are different chants for that particular way to fix it. There are so many songs.

I would use our most basic medicine that covers nearly all; I would use red roots. Old people will ask for red roots because they like the smell of it after it has been sitting there for a couple of days and they're using it for four days. You always put red roots in water. And then there's another one. There is another plant that I would put in there with it. But basically I would use red roots (*mēkko-hoyvnēcv*) because red roots will cover nearly anything internally or externally. That is a basic. That is one of our main medicines.

I would put another plant with it. I would use what we call *kofockv-rakko*. That is one of the basic medicines that we have. We use that to ease your mind. We use red root for the headache, but we use *kofockv-rakko* to ease that person's mind. Maybe she's thinking too much—could be anything. An Indian will go thinking about their bills or their grandkids, what have you. That is one of the best things you can use, *kofockv-rakko*. Lots of times we use that to take a bath. To make the medicine, I would put both of them (*mēkko-hoyvnēcv* and *kofockv-rakko*) in there when I first start. I get my jar and then I put them both in there. And then it really doesn't matter which chant I do first. It doesn't matter, but they are already both together when you get ready to use it.

Then, if their head aches, the chant would depend on the situation. We could have one we think is nothing but stress. Then, say, somebody might have an accident and bump their head. They might be damaged on the inside. They might have done something on the inside causing the headache and it is up to us to decide what we think. And so there are different chants for that headache. It depends on what you think caused the headache. That is why you always listen to them because we don't know if their old man knocked 'em around a few times and then they have a headache, we don't know about it. So we listen to what they are saying and then the more they tell us, the easier for us to help them. If they don't tell us their old man knocked them and they hit their head on the wall, if they don't tell us that part and they tell us something else, then we got to go with what they are telling us and all the time they are leaving the main thing out. We can still help them with their headache, but it would have been a lot easier if they had just come out and said, "I hit my head on a wall."

ARTHRITIS

There are some things that we let them use hot because it gets the job done a lot better by using hot. For arthritis, for example, I make it hot regardless of the weather because the heat will go into the body a lot faster and it draws the pain out, the heat will. But some of them will ask you, will you make that for me where I can use it cold. So you don't argue with them on that, if that is what they want, that's what they get. If it is an arthritis, then the pain itself is one of the basic things because mostly they are complaining it hurts. So that is the thing that we are drawing out, the pain is the main thing that we are concerned with. So you will soak your hand in water but we want you to use it hot so we would use a chant to be hot to draw that pain out. You said it was being caused by arthritis, so now we are using what arthritis would cause. It is causing the pain, but it is caused by arthritis. So there are songs that deal with arthritis causing the pain. Then there are different songs for pain you feel when you fell down and hurt yourself. Let's say that you sprained your wrist or hand. That is an entirely different thing. We would use a pain chant, but then the whole chant itself changes because it is not arthritis, it was caused by a fall. If the arthritis is in your hand, for example, I would probably add something. You know you are going to move it around. We are going to tell you to do that anyway while you are letting it soak. Now if it is beginning to swell, we may add something else to take the swelling down. So we have to see and we have to deal with it as we see fit.

Two of the best things that I think I would use, I would use a cedar and red roots, I would come back to that. If you have got plenty of red roots, I would still stick with the red roots, but if not, cedar is good, darn good. The green part of cedar is used quite a bit in a lot of things, but the only drawback on the cedar is that when placed in water it sours fast. But the red root medicine, you can use that nearly over and over and over again. The old people, they want to use it over and over again even though the color of the water would be just so clear, but they know the medicine is still good. The cedar you cannot use over and over again. It will sour too fast. And they don't use it long before they have got to throw it out.

You always explain what you are going to do anyway and then tell the person how to use it. You will use this four consecutive days. If you miss a day, you start all over again until you make your four days. Especially women, because they may say, well, I am all right, but then they may have their monthly ahead of time and so then that means they have to start again when it is over. Women, the time that they are in their cycle, all the impurities are being expelled out of their body. When they are in that stage there, we don't ever let them take any medicine because it will kill that medicine. It will actually kill the medicine if they try to use it when they are doing that. It is Mother Nature cleaning itself, removing everything. So they can't take medicine because it will take the medicine out also.

That is why the red roots are better because they will last that long. The cedar would never make it. So you would have to throw it out and then go back and get some more. You would probably get two jars of it. The first jar that you get would be marked number one. You use all of that. Okay, then number two, number three is marked on the other jar. All you do is add it to that first one for second day and then third day and fourth day. On the fourth day you combine it all. But you don't ever pour it out. You keep that.[1]

The basic plant is red root. There are backup roots to use if you don't happen to have it. There are always backup roots. You don't have this one, then you have a backup that you can get. Some of them are plentiful in the summertime but would be hard to get in the wintertime, but then you got one that is plentiful that you could have in the wintertime. It is kind of set up where you would have one regardless of the time of the year. So what you rely on, you more or less use the one that is plentiful. If you are using leaves all through the summer, when they fall, then you go back to the roots that you have gathered. And then usually it's red roots; that's your backup. It is your main medicine, but then that is the one that you want to stock up on because it will cover anything that can go wrong with a person.

GUNSHOT WOUNDS

I will tell what Dad said, what he told me, and what Jackson Lewis said about the gunshot wounds. It is probably the hardest of all the chants we have; three things are involved.

Number one, the medicine person is supposed to know how to stop all the bleeding first. The person has to be able to stop the bleeding whether it is just a minor wound or whether it is an artery cut. That is the first thing that the medicine man will have to learn how to do. A man could bleed to death in a minute who is pretty well hit. That is the thing the medicine person has to do first thing. It is not a long chant for that, but you have to work quickly. You would use dirt right off. Your main ingredient would be dirt because you can scoop up the dirt. Not the topsoil itself; you kick that off and get that soil right below it because it is usually moist and you can roll that right into a little ball.

Most likely, if it's out in the open, the medicine person could use dirt. Remember about my dad? My cousin was bleeding, and Dad took a ball of dirt. He made a little ball of dirt. That is all he used, just a little ball of dirt just about the size of a marble. He fixed that, he brought it back and he set it on there. When he removed it, there wasn't a trickle of blood coming out (chapter 5).

The second thing: supposing that a bone was hit, that the person has a lot of splinters or jagged bones that could protrude. The bones that are in there that have been hit and shattered, there is a way to make those things come out, to work themselves out quick, without cutting into it. So anything that will interfere with it healing back, it will work itself out. The medicine person has to know that. They would more likely use the liquid. They would pour liquid medicine on there. You normally would pour it down, if it is a big jagged hole or whatever, you pour it on there. Those are the things you use. Anything that is broken off will work itself out of there; it will come out. The medicine man is not going to stick his hand down in where the man has gotten hit, so he uses medicine to make the bones come back out. The bones will work themselves out. No matter what they are using, if they purify it and put it on there, it will not have an infection set in. It is like when you get a splinter in your hand. You give it enough time and your body's going to push it out. We just move up the process, just speed it up.

It doesn't specify which plants to use. Probably most of the people have red roots with them all the time, no matter where they go. No matter where I go I always have some. All the medicine people always have something with them that they could use in a minute, but the key to everything that we're talking about is the chants. The chants will do it. It doesn't matter what you use if it's from the nature. That is why the pact was made between the man and the plants (chapter 6). We'll do our part. That is why we can reach for pretty near anything and use anything we want and we can still make it work.

And the third important thing that the medicine person has to do is be sure that there will be no infection, no matter what they use. The things that ordinary people would use can get infected. So that is the third thing that the medicine person is supposed to be able to do. No matter what he uses, whether he uses mud, plants, leaves, whatever is handy for him to use and whatever he has, it just depends on where he is and what he has to use. We would more or less use the nature because we trust that more than other things. But no matter what they use, it will not get infected.

Before you pack it, you stop the bleeding, then you get rid of the bone because the medicine that you are making is for that bone to heal. You want that to start getting back together right quick. You can't wait for days and days. There is a story that was told by Jackson Lewis. A person had a big gunshot wound and in four days that man walked off. That was the thing that was done during the Civil War. Back in the old days they used this quite a bit. Close to a creek there are mud and leaves. They probably used that, put it on there to keep air from getting in.

The chants are the key to everything. You make these plants do it. These are long chants on some of these. Some of these are longer than the majority we've got. The thing to keep in mind is there are no set rules on any emergency. We use what is handy. That is why the chants that we have, we can use with nearly anything. Those are the key things. You have chants to make it do what you want it to do, to direct it where you want it to go. People not familiar with our work, they would question some of the things that we use. They may not feel that it would work. But we use what's handy. We know what would work. That is why we fall back upon the nature. We know that the plants will do their part and we do ours. We know they are going to do it. So we use the best thing that we can get our hands on in an emergency. That's what saves lives. We don't have time to run around and go to the store. We have to reach for the ground. So that is the key to the thing that the non-Indians or some of the Indians would have a hard time understanding because they have never seen it. They don't understand. We have no problem with it because we know it works.

MAKING MEDICINE SOAPS

There are so many chants. It never entered my mind how many there would be. Even in fixing a bar of soap like the families use to take a bath with, there are different chants for different things, even soap. There's about thirteen songs that I know just to do one soap. All of them do about the same thing. Some of them can be specific about certain things. But you know my grandmother and my dad, one had six and one had seven songs to do a soap. Some of them, if I haven't used it in a while, I'll throw that song in and use it for a while. Then I'll use a different one next time for a different family. It depends on the situation, too. Say that they feel that somebody has used something against them, against their will. Someone has used negative medicine against them. There are different chants to remove all that. And most of the time, what you do, it really catches all of them anyway because it really purifies the whole body. You remove the negative things. That is why they feel good afterward. It might not be just that anybody did something—you move a lot of the negative things away so they feel good. So it just depends on the situation. You use ginseng root. You scrape that root and it is very, very fine. It is real powdery. Then once you've got that done you cut four slits on your soap and you put the medicine in each. The chants are all done to the medicine itself before it goes into the soap and then once it's in the soap, then you seal it. You can't even see it in the soap if you don't know what you are looking for.

Mostly all the medicine is always sealed. That's why you keep that cover on until you get ready to use it. You say everything four times. You make people use it four times. If they are going to take a bath with it, they all come back every month for the first four months. The old people did that, anyway. Once a year, they all come back to get something and then go home. The old people do; they follow the instructions. They automatically would get it four times. But nowadays it is hard to tell a person. It makes you have a little guilty conscience because it seems like you are telling them to come back. Some of them feel good. They don't think they have to come back again. If they follow the old ways, they come back even if they feel good. It is just a rule, you get it four times, it is just the way it's done.

After you make your fourth time, then that's it. The soap now they take enough to last a long time. If they just take two, then they'll come back again for two more. Make sure you use that four in a row once you start. Some people just like to have it on hand. Those are the ones that live a long, long time. Some of them you do tell them, "You don't need that." But if it's an old person, you don't tell them that. It makes them mad. They'll say, "I want it, that's why I came." So you don't argue with those kind of people. Or they'll say, "Don't you want to make me medicine?" I'll say, "No, it's not that. You came a long ways but you're all right." They will say, "I know what I'm doing. I know what I want." I'll say, "Okay."

One guy, I made soap for him. He watched us put medicine in the soap, but there was doubt in his mind. He cut that soap in two. He couldn't find anything in there. He said, "There's nothing there." Dad took a knife and he cut the other half open and he said, "Look again." The man looked and the powder was all on one side. It was. He said it was strange. Dad said, "You didn't have the belief." They have the way of removing themselves. That guy couldn't find any trace of it. He didn't think we put anything in. And Dad cut that other half up and said, "Look at this." It was just like putting sugar over there piled up. The medicine had all moved to one corner of the bar of soap. We didn't fix him another soap either. We told him to hit the road because he didn't believe enough. That wouldn't have done him any good. We said, "You had a doubt."

I see a lot more old ones than the others. You know that is the odd thing about some of the old people. They are very, very protective of a person, too. You could ask some of them where I live. If they don't know you, they'll tell you they don't even know me. They won't tell you, but they will come to me and tell me someone was asking about you but we told them we didn't know where you live. But if they know you or know of you or know your parents, they will tell you. They are very protective of our medicine. Some people have said they had a hard time finding me because nobody knew me. Even the younger ones do that now. They will look you over, eyeball you good before they open their mouths. They will come tell me, "So and so was asking but we didn't tell them anything."

Most of the old people come after soap for cleansing purpose on the external part and then they'll ask for red roots to throw up to cleanse out the inside. They come at least once a year. They really don't need it, but they have done it all these years and to them it has just got to be done.

THE LITTLE MEASURING CUPS

There are gourds of different sizes and shapes that medicine people gather to be used in the future. Once a gourd is pulled off the vine, it is dried out and stored for a whole year before it is touched again. I can remember my grandmother and I gathering the gourds. I watched her hanging them up in our little smokehouse in the right order that they were to be used. She used the oldest one first, which was to her left as she faced the string of gourds. The newly picked gourd was hung up to the right end of her older gourds. My dad had a small shed close to his house where he hung up his gourds, but there was a time or two he borrowed some small gourd from my grandmother. These gourds gathered were not cut into any shape till they had been seasoned for a minimum of one year. After all the little gourds have been cut to the size and shape needed, they are now ready to be purified. The cedar to be used is doctored; a fire is built and the cedar is put into the fire and stirred around to cause it to smoke. The measuring cup is now held over the smoking fire, purifying it. The last step in purification is to wash all the measuring cups with red root with your hand, washing the inside and outside of the cups. If the gourds have handles on them, you hang them up in a tree, but if there is no handle, you put them on a flat rock. You leave them for a period of four days for all gourds, regardless of any intended purpose. Your measuring cups are now ready to use.

The size and shape of the measuring cup depends on the person that is to use this cup. A small baby usually gets a cup shaped with a spout on it. You can open the baby's lips up and pour the medicine into the little mouth. The little bitty cups that we use are not always for children. The small measuring cups are primarily for medicine that is bitter, regardless of the age of a client. If you give people too much, they are liable to throw up, getting rid of the medicine out of their bodies. So the size of these little measuring gourd cups is according to how much medicine we want a person to take.

Most of our clients that will take medicine over a length of time will get a measuring cup. The medicine person will pour the exact amount of medicine a client will have to take into the cup to show the client. The client is also instructed whether to take the medicine once, twice, or three times a day and at a certain time of the day. I always ask my clients if they understand how much medicine to take, how often and when. If they answer yes to all these questions, I pour that medicine back into the jar and tell them when to start using their medicine.

Cedar for this purification of measuring cups does not have to be a virgin tree, but you always take the cedar from the east side of the tree. We always sing our chants when we are going to touch a tree or collect roots or plants. Remember what the plant said to the young man in the story, "those are the words you will say when you are going to remove us from Mother Earth," and the young man said he would. That is the only time the plant ever gave instructions to a human being and the plant said that from this day on, the medicine people would be known as the keepers of the plants. So, no matter what plant, tree, or roots, it is the same words you say when you take them from the earth. I used the words the plant told the young man to use when even the smallest gourd was pulled off the vine. I know the plants hear me, giving me the right to remove them from Mother Earth.

THE LITTLE HORN

The little horn I use is a cow horn. The story doesn't say what kind of animal we should get our horn from. It could be made from any animal with a horn. To get a horn ready, we go through the same process that we go through for other things, such as our medicine stick. After we get the animal we are going to use, we cut the horn off. After the horn has been cut, it will not be touched for four days. Any time after the first four days, the horn can be cleaned out, the hole can be drilled out from the small end, and the horn can be cut to the length a medicine man desires. The horn is now ready to be purified. The horn is smoked down once a day for a total of four days with medicine using cedar. Once again the horn will be purified using red roots that have been dug fresh. The horn is washed down four times. This type of purification is done once a day for a total of four days in a row before the horn is ready to use.

There are times you use the little horn. One of the times I used my little horn happened during a softball game. There was a team from Seminole and a team from Tulsa in the finals. The batter at the plate was a good hitter. I very seldom had ever seen him get fanned; I watched him many times come to bat in a close game and get a good hit to win the ball game, and I was really rooting for him to hit a home run. He did get a good hit and I thought that would be good enough for a home run because he was also an exceptionally fast runner, but after he came around the second base, he fell down, about halfway between second and third base, and he crawled the rest of the way to third base. He was hurt, so they called time-out and ran to see what happened. I was sitting in the shade watching the game, and they called for me so I went over to them. I could see a big red spot right where he was hurting. I told the coach I needed to go to my car and get something and I would do what I could for his player. I asked the coach if he would help his player walk to the nearby trees, to be away from many watchful eyes. After we got the player behind a big tree, the coach went back to his ball game. I did what is supposed to be done first and using my little horn, I sucked a tail of a scorpion out of his leg. As soon as the scorpion tail was removed, he didn't hurt anymore.

I have also used the horn on people who have been to a clinic and felt they were not getting the right help because their problem was still persistent. If a person hurts in a certain area or spot with a big red ring around it and it really hurts if you just touch it, you usually end up using the little horn. Many Indians will believe someone has put an evil spell on them, but it is not always true. Many of their pains have natural causes, which I have been able to help. There are Creeks and people from other tribes around today who can hurt people. I have many times cut four little bitty cuts around a red sore spot and, using my horn, taken a live fly out of a person's back or shoulder. I'm talking about a big green fly that would fly off if you were to turn it loose.

My family has pulled more spider webs out of people than any other thing. My dad didn't like to do this kind of work because he felt it was women's work. When my grandmother was living, she did most all of this kind of doctoring. Dad and I would only do it if we had no choice. There is an elderly lady still living not too far from me and I don't mind recommending her to some people because she is good in this type of work.

THE TEMPTATON TO USE BAD MEDICINE

Some people are called by other tribes into their areas. People will track down the ones that will do what they want to do. They look for the ones good; they look for the ones bad. People out West now, they are good at hurting people. Clients get their money's worth too; they are really good. They can destroy a person. That's where a lot of people go when they want something real bad to be done. They want something to happen six months from now; they set it up that way. It's hard to trace back because everything will be natural and next thing you know, the person is gone. Everybody wonders what happened. They get their price too. I know one person who went out to look for something like that and he said it cost him forty-five hundred dollars.

I've been offered a brand new sports car, and that was a high-priced car. I said, "No, you are talking to the wrong one." And here I was afoot too. But once you do the bad, you can't come back to the other one, the good. We've always looked at it that way. You would never be effective anymore. Day by day, the things you could have done good are taken away from you. That is why a main *heles-hayv* walks a fine line. If greed beats you, if you may think, "Oh, it's not going to hurt them all that bad," you just crossed the line. You broke everything that you were given in trust. Your teachers gave you their power, but they will also take it back. You could lose it by misusing it. Usually what happens is the person who misuses it would probably just go ahead and continue the bad way. They get good at it too. But they would never cure again. They may do it, they may make the medicine, but it would never do any good. All they are doing is going through a routine. When they initiate you they say all the things that you will be able to do, but they also add that if you misuse that, the power they gave you will be taken back. You will no longer have that power.

Your instructors had to teach you both ways because, from the beginning, there will always be good; there is always bad. You learn both ways. I was very fortunate that I had some strong people train me. You couldn't tempt them to hurt anybody. I mean, they were good. One reason that I would never do the bad is that they had so much faith in me that they were willing to give me their power. Just knowing that alone will keep you from doing anything wrong because if you do, you are letting them down. I would be letting down my grandma and my dad and medicine people further back, way, way back, who passed the medicine down. If you do the bad, you just destroyed it all. I would never do that. It came this far. I don't want to destroy it by being greedy.

Chapter Nine

CEREMONIES

I was asked to do a blessing to the old Creek Nation Council House early in the morning. This building belongs to the city of Okmulgee, Oklahoma, but the tribe may try to get it back. The blessing has never been done at the Council House for probably a hundred years, so they wanted a blessing there. The majority of the Mvskoke people have never seen a blessing take place. The last time one was done was in 1966. I've only seen one done twice in my lifetime.

THE BLESSING CEREMONY
In doing the blessing, the main medicine man or any medicine person always has an assistant. Normally I could have used one assistant, but I used two that day. The two assistants I chose were my choice because of their strong belief in our medicine ways. The fire keeper chosen was a medicine man and supreme court judge of the Creek Nation. The second chosen assistant was a Creek Nation tribal court judge.

Preparing Medicines
Let me tell you about the materials that were used during the blessing, starting with the wood for the fire. Let me explain why I was thrilled to be asked to do the blessing that day. Once again I was working with my dad in spirit, and his work once again was going to be used. The firewood used was gathered and doctored by my dad and me working together to be used someday in the future, and that was over twenty-five years ago.

It is very hard to find a fallen tree for our purpose because of grass fires burning up the trees. There are many hours spent walking and looking for a dead tree that was once healthy and died of old age. When I was walking with Dad, I carried the stuff and he just walked and we looked. Dad and I found many dead trees that seemed like good ones but as we tested one, it turned out a lightning had once struck that tree, causing it to die. You must prepare yourself physically and mentally using medicine for just that purpose. You also carry the medicine to be used to test the fallen tree to see if it is fit to use. When we found a dead tree that met our approval, it was sprinkled down or "washed" with another medicine, using two fingers dipped into that medicine to sprinkle. We purified it and then we brought it back, and that is when we really went to work on it. The gathered wood is doctored to be used for a blessing. The prepared wood must also be wrapped tight to avoid having the sacred words escape. So Dad and I prepared that firewood years ago to be used only in a blessing.

Let me tell you about the cedar that is used for a blessing. A medicine man spends hours in the woods walking, looking, and trying to locate a young "virgin tree" that will fit his purpose for what he is to perform. Once a medicine man feels he has located what will meet his needs, he will walk away from that tree, never touching it until he comes back another day. When we talk about a virgin tree, we are talking about a young tree standing about five or six feet tall and that has never been touched by a human being. Once again the medicine man prepares himself and the medicine to test the cedar tree to see if this is the tree to use. You use medicine on your hands and face and then you can go up, walk up to a tree like that and put your hand on there and run your hand up through there and you can tell if that tree has ever been touched by another human being because you will get different feedback. You'll find the spot where they touched. When your hand goes up from the bottom of the tree, you'll stop right on the spot. This tree's been touched by another human being. Then we leave that tree alone and we go to another one. This so-called special cedar tree to a medicine man doesn't always work out, so he goes to other trees he has located, testing, as he continues to look for the one he will use. Once a virgin tree is found, a medicine man will double-check, making sure this is a virgin tree by checking all four sides of the tree, starting from the north side, starting from the bottom of the tree with his hands going upward to the top of the tree. West, south, east sides of the tree are checked the same way as the north side. A medicine man is getting a feedback from that young tree as he puts his hands on it. After all the hard work, preparing, locating a tree, the medicine man will clip only enough cedar for his purpose from the east side of that tree and never use that cedar tree again.

For the blessing, I also prepared other medicines. I prepared tobacco for feeding the fire. I made two liquid medicines, one for purification to sprinkle myself and my assistants before entering the sacred ground and a second one for sprinkling all those who would enter the building for the blessing ceremony. I also prepared a cedar and sage tied together to use in blessing the building.

Setting up the Sacred Ground

I had put four medicine poles in the ground outside the council house building long before the blessing began.[1] This was done for purification of the ground for that day only. All the main medicine people are required to have a sacred ground. There are many hours spent selecting sacred poles and many more hours preparing medicine that would be put into the sacred poles and capped. I use water reed for the poles, but it doesn't have to be water reed. To put the medicine in the pole you can hollow out the inside of what will be the top side of the pole and put it in and cap it off with wood or another natural material. Water reeds are divided into sections with joints in between and when you use water reed, you can put a hole in one of the sections and put the medicine in and then fill in the hole.

The feathers that will be tied to the sacred poles take much longer to prepare because before one can be tied to a sacred pole, the feather is doctored for four days straight. So to prepare four feathers takes sixteen days. We always use feathers. The birds were given the responsibility to take care of the plants, to kind of oversee them, let them know the changing of time. I am glad I am a Bird Clan because anything with the feather, we treasure. We respect those things. The bird has its purpose on this earth and that was given a long, long time ago. He plays a very important part in what we do. Once a medicine man puts his sacred poles into the ground forming a square, the removing of all things that are negative from the ground inside the square continues working until the medicine man removes the poles from the ground. That is because the medicine poles kill out everything negative inside the square. The only time a medicine man will ever remove his medicine poles is to move them to another place he has chosen. Once doctored, the sacred poles of that medicine man will never be doctored again because these sacred poles are his and his alone, never to be passed on to another person.

A medicine man must take his time in selecting a place he will call his sacred ground. The one he uses all the time will be out in the woods. This sacred ground chosen will be where all the most important action will take place in his lifetime. A sacred square is where all the medicine people would go and sit to communicate with their Creator and strengthen their sacred words. Also all the burdens of other peoples that the medicine people have treated that are now on the shoulders of the medicine people are removed once the medicine people step into their sacred grounds. You now have an idea of the purpose of the sacred poles.

I made a sacred ground outside the council house that day. At the blessing, I put the four poles in the ground and spread a blanket inside them. A sacred fire will also be lit inside the square made by the four poles. The blanket in the square had four items laid out on it, one being an eagle feather, another a medicine stick, and the others two small gourds. A medicine of cedar and sage is used to do the actual blessing. When the cedar and sage medicine is lit to do the blessing on the outside and inside of the building, the eagle feather is to be used for fanning the smoke to go the direction you want it to go. The medicine stick was used when I was preparing the medicines. It is still involved with what was laid before us. The stick is very seldom ever left out of anything. The gourd lying on the blanket on the right as you face east contains tobacco for the purpose of feeding the sacred fire. Any time a medicine man uses a fire that will have a direct effect on medicine roots and sacred words, the medicine man will always give thanks and feed the sacred fire. From that fire we will light our cedar and sage to bless the building. The gourd on the left contains cedar from a virgin tree. The cedar is poured on the fire about the same time the tobacco is being applied and the cedar causes the fire to smoke. The cedar from the gourd is to let our Creator know that a blessing has begun and for him to look down and be with us as I do our work.

The Work of the Assistants

The two assistants chosen have two specific things to do. The first assistant's job is to sprinkle the medicine man with the medicine for purification just before he enters the sacred square, even though he really doesn't need this because a medicine man is always ready to enter a sacred square that he has prepared. The medicine man will then sprinkle his assistant or assistants, allowing them to enter the sacred square to build a fire. The second thing the first assistant will do is to sprinkle the medicine man with another medicine that has been prepared to use on those entering the building chosen for the blessing. Once again the medicine man will sprinkle his assistant or assistants, allowing them to enter the building, but the assistant will stand by the door and sprinkle all the people who are entering the building and will be the last person to enter the building and close the door so that the blessing can begin. The medicine used to sprinkle the medicine man and his assistants before they enter the sacred ground is a different medicine from the one used to sprinkle the medicine man, his assistants, and all the others who enter the building to be blessed.

The second assistant is to build a fire, and he could also assist the first assistant. The fire man has two primary purposes. He builds the fire with wood that has been prepared for the blessing. As the fire begins to blaze, he will put lots of prepared cedar into the fire, causing it to smoke. The smoke from the sacred fire is to purify the air of all negative things or negativity that is around the place that is to be blessed and at the same time to let the Creator know the sacred blessing is about to begin so he may look down and watch and bless us in our work. The fire man's second job is to see that the fire doesn't go out while all the basic things are being done.

Calling on the Creator and the
Medicine People of Yesterday

To start the ceremony, the medicine man and the assistants are sprinkled. Purifying the body itself is one thing, but at that same time the medicine man is giving the assistant permission to handle anything that he's got. And also the assistant has the authority or permission to step into the square. I sprinkled them both. That is the only time that they were allowed to step in the square. At any other time they wouldn't be. They entered the square and the fire man started the fire. Then I poured the tobacco and the cedar on the fire. As you pour the tobacco and cedar on the fire, you repeat some of the words that were told to you during your training about how the blessing ceremony is to be performed. It has been told that our Creator will always help our people. These are the words of the old medicine people of my family:

> Creator, I am calling on you now.
> Creator, you have given us sacred words to use.
>   I am using it now.
> Creator, you have instructed us to involve all of our medicine people
>   of yesterday, I am calling them now.
> Creator, I have opened the heaven's door for all to join us
>   in our sacred blessing.

Once you put the cedar on the fire, the thing smokes and the smoke starts going up and it is to let our Creator know that we are ready to do our work. What we are doing, we are telling our Creator, we let him know that our work has begun, that he may smile down on us and be with us for that particular work. In all the blessings that you do, you are required to involve all the people of yesterday; all the medicine people of yesterday you are calling back. In your mind you are visualizing them all coming back. You can feel them all coming back. So you give them time; they are gathering. You are opening the door wide for them. That is one beautiful thing about this because you can feel the energy. That day my arms, the hairs on my arms, they all just popped up, straight out. The energy was coming back; they were gathering, you could tell. You have to go through that and you know then that you did it right. My dad, my grandma and my great grandpa, it was just like they were looking down on me: "Hey, he's going to do the blessing." That is one beautiful thing about our ways. Those people of yesterday are never forgotten. That's why they said, "We will always be there." And then when we start doing something, you want them also to be there. That is why we gather them back. That is a good feeling to know that they are involved—beautiful feeling, a really good feeling.

Blessing the Building

All the basic requirements had been finished. Now the medicine that was the cedar and sage tied together was put to the sacred fire to start it to burn so the blessing could begin. Cedar and sage in the one hand and eagle feather in the other hand, the medicine man and his assistants leave the sacred square and go to the north side of the building that is to be blessed. The medicine man and his assistants now stand facing the building, with the medicine man holding the cedar and sage and the eagle feather to fan the smoke toward the building. The north side completed, the medicine man and his assistants go, moving counterclockwise, to the west side, repeating the same procedure as at the north side. Having completed the west side, once again moving counterclockwise they go to the south side, repeating the same procedure as on the north and west sides. After completing the south side they go to the east side and repeat the same procedure. The four sides of the building have now been smoked. You always end in the east because the east is a new day, a new life. The medicine on each side of the building will now move toward the center of the building, connecting and completing a circle around the building.

The blessing on the outside is completed and the medicine man and his assistants now go to the entrance of the building. The assistant sprinkles the medicine man with the sacred medicine and the medicine man also sprinkles his assistants before they enter the building. One of the assistants then sprinkles the people that may want to enter. This assistant will be the last person to enter the building, closing the door. Once inside the building, the medicine man may start with any room he chooses. Once he has decided, he will smoke each corner of that room, going counterclockwise. He needs to do this in the room only once. After completing a room he goes to another room, moving counterclockwise, smoking each corner of that room. This procedure is followed until all the rooms of the building are completed. He only needs to do the downstairs rooms because the medicine will reach the upstairs rooms.

The blessing of the building is now completed; the medicine man will go back out to the sacred ground, put out the fire, and pick up his sacred poles. He picks them up counterclockwise and secures them in a tight container. All the words that we use are alive, so anytime that we move these poles around, when we pick them up and move them from the ground, we always put them in a capped container so that the words will never get away. They will stay within the medicine itself. All the medicines that are made are done that way. We always cap these things. As he picks each stick up he points it in the four directions and up and down in recognition of the directions and the Creator and Mother Earth. You are just giving thanks. The ceremony is over.

DOCTORING A HOUSE

The procedures for doctoring a house and for blessing a place are similar; yet they are different in many ways. When doctoring a house, the medicine man does not prepare a sacred ground or need an assistant. He builds his own fire in a bucket or some type of container. He puts cedar and tobacco on the fire, causing it to smoke; he will now go around the building four times, going counterclockwise. That is different from the blessing because in the blessing, you only go around the building once, but you make four stops. When doctoring a house, once the outside is finished to his satisfaction, the medicine man will go into the house, starting with any room he chooses, he will smoke out each room going counterclockwise until all the rooms have been smoked four times. Doctoring a house does not require a medicine man to smoke four corners of each room like in the blessing, but he may do so if he wants to do it. He does walk through each room four times. In the blessing, he only goes through each room once.

Another way to doctor a house is to have a medicine man prepare some cedar and tobacco, giving it to the homeowners to smoke out the house themselves and following his instructions as to who in the family should do it and when to do it. He might tell them to do it way in the night or early in the morning, for example.

These are just a few reasons why medicine people are called to doctor a house: When people feel something is making them uneasy about their place, they might call. It could be a strange noise that doesn't seem normal to them. There could be lots of sickness in their family, which they believe should not be happening, or lots of bad luck to that family. Most often the reason to get a house doctored is hearing noise in the house. Noise heard could be dishes moving around in the kitchen sink for unknown reasons, a door opening when no one is there, someone in the room causing the wooden floor to squeak when no one is there to be seen, or water buckets being moved around, hearing people dipping in there to get water out. These few things I mention cause many children and adults to be afraid in their own homes.

The medicine man's job is to get rid of these kinds of problems for the families who seek his help. If there is sickness and they feel there is bad luck there, you can remove all of those things. But, as far as removing the people that come back and can be heard walking, I don't ever recommend for them to remove that from the house because once we remove that, they won't ever hear these sounds again. It could be their loved ones coming back. And then once you remove it, they'll never hear these sounds again. Last time I did something like that, I tried to talk this guy out of doing it, but he said the kids were getting scared and he wanted it done. I said, well, it won't be just a few years off they'll grow up and leave, but you will always be here. But he insisted I go ahead and remove all the things from the house. I did. Now he is sorry about it because there is nothing I can do. He wants to hear those sounds that he used to hear so you know they're back, you hear them walking around, moving chairs. Those kind of sounds, I like to hear them.

There is also an entirely different thing for a house if you want the past loved ones to stay and always be there—so that it would be easy for them to stay and come back. In this one you are not removing anything negative, but you could remove things negative that were there. What you are doing is removing anything that would ever interfere with that energy for the person to be welcome to come back. There is nothing keeping them from coming back. They are welcome to stay, come back anytime they want. It is almost the same procedure that you would use in doctoring a house. The chants are different. We have songs for just about everything that could ever be thought of.

REBURIAL

This is the story my great grandfather, Jackson Lewis, told my dad. He said to Dad that this is something that someday you might have to use. Maybe you never will, but there is a possibility. These are the procedures to follow and the sacred words to be used before a grave is opened up to move the remains to another location for reburial.

For some strange reason Dad said to me,

> I knew he [Jackson Lewis] wasn't going to talk about our graves around here. I could sense his feeling as he started talking about his bad experience as a young man. Your great grandfather stressed the importance of neutralizing the ground at the grave sites. His main reason for talking about neutralizing the ground was that during the removal, a lot of our people lost their spouses, children, friends, and loved ones. There were powerful medicine people among them and they were very bitter and hurt about what was taking place to

our people. Every time they would lose one of their people, a medicine man would doctor the deceased's belongings to hurt whoever
opened up that grave by releasing the bad medicine that was on the
belongings of the deceased, no matter when it took place.

The medicine people geared this type of bad medicine toward the non-
Indians who would more likely dig into the graves of our people. The
medicine was not only to hurt those persons who opened the grave but
their families as well. They knew there was a slim chance of an Indian
getting hurt because of their respect for the deceased. Indians would never
open a grave, but they could be hurt also if they should ever dig into the
graves that had been doctored. Anything that Indians used or had, their
belongings and equipment, the others wouldn't take away from them when
they died. They would put everything in the grave. The non-Indians don't
put anything in the graves, but Indians load them down. Now, another
Indian will never want to fool with that grave, but the non-Indians, they
would dig into anything. So in order to get back at the non-Indians during
the removal, the medicine people did do a lot of things to the belongings
so that these would affect the person who was fooling with the grave and
that person's family. So that's why my great grandfather talked about
neutralizing the ground before moving a grave.
    My great grandfather gave Dad these procedures for him to follow if
he was ever called on to move the remains of the deceased from one burial
place to another for reburial. The first procedure is to let the people select
the medicine man who is to be in charge, who is to make the medicine.
So the tribe has the say-so in who they pick. Then the medicine man, in
turn, selects an assistant to carry out his instruction. The assistant then
will select others to help him. This medicine man first prepares himself
to handle any unknown problem that may occur. He does a lot of soul
searching. He has to be sure these people who are going to be selected
will follow his instructions and keep his sacred words holy. The assistant
that the medicine man selects must be dedicated to his work because of
the type of responsibility he has to carry out in this important task. The
assistant is responsible for putting medicine out for neutralizing a grave
site but also must pick a person to be "mouth" or "speaker" and must
pick the grave diggers if the remains have to be dug.
    After the people for this important mission have been handpicked, the
medicine man must prepare medicine to purify their bodies, internally and
externally, so that they will be physically and mentally ready long before
their journey begins. He makes medicine to clean them out. Their bodies
and minds are already prepared once they get on the road to go wherever

the graves are, so that when they get there, they are ready to go through the procedure of removing. After arrival at their destination, the medicine man makes medicine for neutralizing the grave site or where the remains are located and he has his assistant put out the medicine according to his instructions. The assistant has the medicine, probably in dry form, in a gourd and spreads it on the ground around the graves. The medicine will work its way to the center of the grave. You can put it on the grave too, but all you need is to put it around the grave. The assistant only has to put this medicine out once.

The next procedures involve the deceased. The medicine man makes medicine to call back the spirits of the deceased so that they can be there with the living as they go through the procedure of removing the remains from their resting place. This procedure involves the living and the deceased and it is carried out by the "mouth" or speaker. For four days, each morning before the sun comes up, the speaker washes with the medicine that has been prepared especially for him. Then at sunrise he makes his first round walking around the graves. He could just walk around the graves once at that time, but more than likely he will walk around them four times. If I were doing it I would walk around them four times. Then during the day he will make three more rounds around the graves. The speaker will make four rounds around the graves during the day, each day, but will use his medicine only once in the early morning of each of the four days, and his first round each day will be at sunrise. He might make his other rounds at ten, at three, and six, or whenever he wants and in between he can walk and talk at the graves when he wants. He will go counterclockwise around the graves as he does this work. The speaker talks to the remains over and over again.

The speaker's job is to explain to the spirits that they have been called back to their graves, that their remains are going to be removed from the ground and taken back to where their people are located now. The speaker is getting their cooperation. The speaker is to talk to the remains and spirits over and over, explaining why their resting place is being disturbed and the good part—that they are to be reunited with their loved ones. It would be just like talking to another person. In other words, just like a conversation, just as if you were talking to them.

The last procedure is the selection of grave diggers. The one that the main medicine man has selected as his assistant must select the grave diggers he is comfortable with, which can be any number of people he feels will be needed to dig the grave or to remove the remains from any institution that has the remains in storage. The medicine man makes the medicine for his assistant to use with the grave diggers. The grave diggers stand facing east at the grave site. The assistant sprinkles the face of each digger with the medicine as the diggers stand facing the east and the assistant walks around the diggers four times. The grave diggers start using their medicine at the same time the speaker is using his medicine, each morning before the sun rises. There is a difference between the speaker and grave diggers in how many times the medicine is used. You must remember the speaker only uses his medicine once a day but will go around the grave four times each day in sets of four, making sixteen rounds total in four days. At the same time the speaker is going around, the grave diggers are to be sprinkled in their faces by the assistant with the medicine made especially for them. The assistant sprinkles them first and then the assistant makes his first four rounds around all his diggers, who are standing facing east. This now makes this one complete round. The assistant will once again sprinkle the faces of the diggers and walk around them four times again, completing the second round. The third and fourth rounds follow the same procedure as the first and second, which now makes four complete rounds. In each of the four rounds, the assistant sprinkles the diggers only once but he walks around them four times. The diggers will be sprinkled sixteen times and the assistant will have walked around them sixty-four times in four days.

The last day of using their medicine is very important. Every day it is done at sunrise, but the one that is the key to the whole thing is the last one. It is so important that all the people that are involved have to watch the sun rise each day after they have arrived at their location. They are watching the sun rise each day so that they can time their last day of taking their medicine to coincide with the sunrise as nearly as possible. So that as the sun begins to come up, that's when the assistant sprinkles the faces of the grave diggers for the last round of the last day. They will time the sunrise on their watches to see what time it is each morning; this is done in case it is cloudy on the fourth day. The sunrise symbolizes something that is very important to Indians on a special occasion such as this kind of work we medicine people do. We know the spirits will once again rise to join us for a little while. The assistant and the diggers watch the sun as it is just breaking daylight, just beginning to come over the mountain or wherever they are, just as it is beginning to peek. That is when they do the last set of rounds. If it was the fourth day and it did not work out, if they did not do it at sunrise, they would have to go through the whole procedure from the beginning.

After that is done, then the grave diggers can dig up the remains. The grave diggers' job is completed once they remove the remains from the grave or remove the remains from where they are stored. Now, the speaker will stay with the remains until they reach their new location and must

talk to the remains as they travel home. There is no set time or require-
ment for how many times he is to talk to the remains as they travel. The
speaker will always stay with the remains as they travel. In other words,
he is always around close; he is never away from the remains very long.
The speaker is the only one who can talk to the remains. When they reach
the new grave site, the jobs of the medicine man, assistant, speaker, and
grave diggers are now completed. The people that are going to dig the
new grave will have done it and the remains will be buried in a normal
funeral that we have at our churches.

The medicine man is always there during the whole procedure of
removal. He will have the medicines ready as they are needed. All he
does is prepare the medicine for them to use. His assistant is the one who
puts all these medicines down; that is the assistant's job. It seems like the
speaker has a big job because he has to stay with the remains and continue
to talk to them. If I were the speaker reburying ones from the removal,
probably the thing that I would do is that I would explain that the place
that the people are buried wasn't their choice. Our people left them behind
because there was no choice. Now the time has come to rejoin their loved
ones and we have a place for them. It is their choice whether to come back
and join us and be once again with our people. I would say, "Our love
for our people is so great, so this is why we are coming to take you back
home with us and all we need is your cooperation, that you follow us in
spirit back to your new resting place." I would continue explaining that
the place where they are buried, there was just no choice then, but they
now have a choice to go and let their spirits flow among our people and
join the other spirits of our people that have passed on in this new land
where we now live. So I would tell them, "Let us gather up your remains
and let's all go home together to where you really belong, with our people
and it will be your new location. Your remains will be there. That will be
your place from now on." After they are reburied, I would thank them for
their cooperation because once you put them in the ground, they don't
want to be disturbed. Then I would probably tell them, "Welcome home.
You are back home. Now rest in peace."

If you were reburying remains from a museum, you would perform
the whole thing. Everything. If I was doing it, I would go to the museum.
The ritual would take place right in that building, right where they are. I
wouldn't let them move anything out of there until I do it. You wouldn't
want to remove them without going through the ritual. I would ask the
museum people to leave the remains alone. Don't fool with them and let
us do our thing. We'll take it from there. I think they would be courteous
enough to let you do that. That's our way.

Chapter Ten

THE UNSEEN POWERS
OF TRADITIONAL MEDICINE

All medicines came from organic sources. Modern medicine now uses synthetic drugs to imitate some of these organic medicines.

The so-called primitive human societies had medicines for their people. Associated with the herbal medicines was what is called conjuring. This is what the modern culture calls it, and it has been dispelled as superstition. What the modern educated man fails to recognize is that there are a great many things that he does not know that are in the unseen worlds of creation.

Modern medicine seems to be limited to powers of the physical and the material. I believe in the so-called primitive way that recognizes powers beyond the visible and beyond man's so-called smart thinking. The modern material world studies and analyzes mainly what can be seen. The ancient traditional recognized the unseen source of what is seen and this is what most people today have been *trained not to see.*

The ancient traditional recognizes and is trained to know about this from the very beginning of the learning. These are powers, energies, intelligence; what is known by the medicine people is not a complex knowledge of time-consuming chemical analysis. It is a simple but sacred impartation to a recipient who is prepared to receive.

The power lies in a total respect toward the tasks of fasting, cleansing, prayer words and creation. Words that come from the energy worlds are simple and known by the medicine people. The original instruction to us stated: "I will come half the way, then you must come half the way."

In other words, creation is here for us to use, not to misuse, not to conquer. It is half the way, for it already has *its* powers, energies, and intelligence. We humans must align ourselves through fasting, prayer, and taking the cleansing medicines to come half the way with all respect, for it is sacred. For the Indians, the words have already been told and are to be passed along but with the same preparation. By this we do our part and come half the way. This is like an agreement with creation and when we do this, we are in harmony and can have good success.

Materialism has disrupted many things that were for the good of all human beings. Materialism is the aggressive, egotistical brainchild of human beings who have forgotten the intelligent, passive gifts of the unseen creation. If we are to do the *complete* good, we must harmonize ourselves, make ourselves sensitive to the powers, energies, and influences of creation. The so-called primitive conjuring of powers, in use with herbal medicines among the native people of this land, still lives.

Appendices

Ann T. Jordan

APPENDIX A

Mvskoke Medicine and the Written Record

David Lewis's account of Mvskoke medicine is a valuable contribution to the written record. In these appendices his account is placed in the context of that record by reviewing those descriptions of medicine and religion already committed to the written tradition. An appropriate place to begin is with an overview of the authors who have written on Mvskoke medicine and the historical and cultural contexts of their work. This is presented in appendix A. The authors' references to topics Lewis discusses are correlated with Lewis's chapters and presented in appendix B. This arrangement contextualizes Lewis's narrative within the written record of Mvskoke religious tradition.

As a sacred tradition transmitted orally, Mvskoke medicine information has rarely been committed to writing by its practitioners. Just as with Mvskoke history, written information about medicine is authored primarily by non-Mvskoke. Prior to removal in the 1830s, the record was provided mostly by traders, government agents, naturalists, and soldiers, who recorded easily observable aspects of Mvskoke religion—everyday rituals like the taking of the black drink or the elaborate annual Green Corn Ceremony. These references to religion were usually brief; the bulk of writings pertained to the magnificent resources of the country and the political and military strength or weakness of the Mvskoke Confederacy vis-à-vis the writer's own government's forces.

The written record after removal is more focused on the recording of culture and religion. This is partly due to the formation of the Bureau of American Ethnology by the United States government in the late nineteenth century. The purpose of this organization was to record information about American Indian cultures. The recording was conducted by trained, non-Mvskoke ethnographers (anthropologists). Others who began to record information were the Mvskoke themselves. They presented a different perspective from the more numerous outsider accounts. In this appendix the intent and perspective of important Mvskoke and non-Mvskoke chroniclers is described along with an accounting of the type of information they recorded. In order to place the written record in historical context, the record is explained here using the same chapter subheadings used in chapter 1 of this book. This review demonstrates how little Mvskoke medicine is understood by non-Mvskoke and how any interpretation of information is just that: an interpretation by an author (whether Mvskoke or non-Mvskoke) whose perspective is colored by his or her own worldview and interests.

THE FUR TRADE YEARS, 1700–1800

The English began settling the colony of Georgia in 1733, and in 1735 an account involving religion was presented by a Mvskoke leader. This is Tchikilli's well-known presentation to Governor Oglethorpe of the Georgia Colony. At Savannah, Tchikilli presented Oglethorpe a buffalo skin on which a migration legend was depicted. Tchikilli told the legend; it was translated into English, and the original skin and translation were later lost. What survives is a German translation of the same. The depictions on this skin describe the migration of the people of Cusseta (Kasihta) from the West into the Southeast and include references to the origins of several medicine plants. While these plants were used in Cusseta, one cannot know whether they were used in all the independent *tvlwv* or by all medicine people.[1]

In the years following Tchikilli's presentation, several Europeans visited Mvskoke towns and recorded information on religion. They included Thomas Nairne, a native of Scotland who served as an Indian agent for the colony of South Carolina and who was later killed in the Yamasee War; James Adair, also a Scot who resided in South Carolina and served as an Indian agent, but who made his living primarily from the trade in deerskins; James Bosomworth, an Indian agent for South Carolina, whose wife, Mary Bosomworth, was of Mvskoke descent and spoke Mvskoke; Jean-Bernard Bossu, a French naval officer who visited the Mvskoke as part of his duties in the French colony of Louisiana; and Hall, an Englishman who visited the Mvskoke as an emissary from the governor of East Florida. With the exception of James Adair, the references these individuals made to Mvskoke religion in their writings were for the most part about the taking of the black drink in the square in several *tvlwv* and about the Green Corn Ceremony. Their primary interest in the Mvskoke was in negotiating with them for European political and economic interests.[2]

Adair, however, was a studious observer of Indian life and in 1775 published a history of the American Indians. Adair's reports on Indian religion were more detailed than those of the others. His writings were influenced by his belief that the American Indians were the descendants of the lost tribes of Israel, a thesis he attempted to prove in his accounting of Indian culture. As is the case with all these early chroniclers, Adair exhibited a Eurocentric bias regarding the Indians. He wrote, "Our rules ought not to allow so mischievous and dangerous a body as the Muskohge to engross this vast forest, mostly for wild beasts. . . . [We must defeat] this haughty nation . . . or drive them over the Mississippi."[3] While Adair provided much cultural data on the Indians of the Southeast, he frequently did not distinguish the cultural data by tribe but rather mixed all the southeastern tribes together. His specific section on the Mvskoke did little to describe their culture and the variations among the *tvlwv*. Instead it was an assessment of their political strength and position vis-à-vis the colonists. His suggestion that the Mvskoke be driven west of the Mississippi seems an ominous foreshadowing of what was to happen to this powerful nation approximately half a century later.

In the years just before and during the American Revolution, one of the important chroniclers of eighteenth-century Mvskoke life was traveling the interior. William Bartram, a Quaker and an English traveler, naturalist, and writer, visited the Mvskoke between 1773 and 1776. Bartram romanticized the Mvskoke, possibly in order to criticize that in contemporary European life which offended his Quaker values.[4] Bartram's work included numerous references to Mvskoke culture and religion. He described his understanding of their concept of a Great Spirit, which was the "Giver and Taker Away of the Breath of Life"; of their belief in shamanic powers to change the weather and cure sickness; of their religious specialists, whom he described as the "High Priest and Juniors in every Town or Tribe"; of their belief in an afterlife and in the soul; of their description of the busk, or "first fruits feast"; and of their descriptions of plants used as medicines, including their botanical names.[5] This detail by a sympathetic author is one of the most valuable of the eighteenth-century outsider sources. Characteristic of his perspective is this passage:

> I know that a Creek Indian would not only receive in his house a Traveler or Sojourner of whatever Nation, color or Language, . . . and here treat him as a Brother . . . as long as he pleases to Stay, and this without the least hope or thought of interest or reward, but serves you with the best of every thing his ability can afford.[6]

Bartram shared his knowledge of the southeastern Indians with the leaders of the young American republic. His written works began to appear in 1791, about the time Alexander McGillivray declared himself leader of the Mvskoke.

McGillivray played a role not only in Mvskoke politics but in the lasting records of Mvskoke culture and religion. Because McGillivray was three-quarters European in descent, other Europeans desiring to be active in the Mvskoke area attached themselves to him. At the same time that Bartram was traversing the Southeast, a Frenchman named LeClerc Milfort arrived in America. Being interested in American Indians, he set out for the interior and found himself in Coweta, one of the Mvskoke *tvlwv*, in 1776. There he met Alexander McGillivray, and the two became allies. Milfort married one of McGillivray's sisters and was an active supporter of McGillivray's political activities. Milfort eventually declared himself *Tastanegy (tvstvnvke)*, or "Great War Chief" of the Mvskoke nation during the years McGillivray was declaring himself the leader of the Mvskoke.[7] When McGillivray was forced to flee Mvskoke lands for fear of his life after the signing of the Treaty of New York, Milfort followed. Without McGillivray's protection, Milfort felt his own life was in danger. Eventually Milfort returned to France and wrote a memoir in which he made references to Mvskoke religion. He referred to the drinking of the black drink and to the Green Corn "harvest" festival.[8] Although he lived for many years among the Mvskoke, his writings suggest that he had little knowledge of religion. He commented, for example, on "the savages having no other religious ceremonies than the taking of the war medicine, which is performed by a kind of doctor."[9]

McGillivray was accompanied back from the signing of the Treaty of New York by Caleb Swan. Swan was primarily interested in describing the vast resources in the Mvskoke lands to United States officials. Swan subsequently submitted a report to Henry Knox, the U.S. secretary of war. He described Mvskoke country in glowing terms, considered its inhabitants lazy for not putting the land to better use, and coveted the land for Euro-Americans.

> The surrounding country [going up the Alabama River toward Little Tallassie] is well watered; the soil is of a dark brown color, with deep strata of red and brown clay, and with the slovenly management even of the savages, it produces most abundantly.... At present it [the country claimed by the Creeks] is but a rude wilderness, exhibiting many natural beauties, which are only rendered unpleasant by being in possession of the jealous natives. The country ... must, in process of time, become a most delectable part of the United States.[10]

As with many of the Europeans and Euro-Americans who eyed Mvskoke land over the centuries, Swan considered the land in its natural, uncultivated state as unused and empty, though from a Mvskoke perspective it was in use for hunting territory and was of spiritual or religious significance. Swan's account provides much information on religion. He described funeral rituals, the black drink ceremony, diseases, medicine cures and medicine people, and ceremonial dances. His reports include a description of the Green Corn Ceremony with McGillivray's name recorded at the end, leading one to suspect that this description was given to Swan by his host. It is not clear that Swan actually witnessed this event. Swan's account of religion remains one of the most detailed of the eighteenth century.[11]

Benjamin Hawkins, the U.S. agent who worked to acculturate the Mvskoke from 1796 to 1816, recorded valuable details about Mvskoke life. Unlike Milfort, who spent years with the Mvskoke but was primarily interested in political power and uninterested in cultural detail, Hawkins focused on Mvskoke culture. This focus was important to his goal of acculturating the Mvskoke. His "Sketch of Creek Country" was read by later chroniclers of Mvskoke culture like Woodward, Stiggins, and Pickett and possibly was used to augment their own understanding of Mvskoke life. His work has been used by most ethnohistorians of the Mvskoke since. He described the Green Corn Ceremony, the making of medicine, medicine plants, the ceremony initiating youth into manhood, the afterlife, and the black drink.[12] Of the Green Corn Ceremony, Hawkins contributes a description that recognizes variation among the *tvlwv*:

This annual festival is celebrated in the months of July or August. The precise time is fixed by the Mic-co and counselors, and is sooner or later, as the state of the affairs of the town, or the early or lateness of their corn, will suit for it. In Cussetuh [Cusseta], this ceremony lasts for eight days. In some towns of less note, it is but four days.... This happy institution of the *Boos-ke-tuh* restores man to himself, to his family and to his nation. It is a general amnesty, which not only absolves the Indians from all crimes, murder only excepted, but seems to bury guilt itself in oblivion.[13]

Plants that Hawkins mentions include *miko hoyanidja* (*mēkko-hoyvnēcv*), *hilis hacinatki* (*heles-hvtke*), *wilana* (*welanv*), *atcina* (*vcenv*) and *pasa* (*passv*).[14]

THE RED STICK WAR AND
INCREASING LAND PRESSURE, 1800–1836

Hawkins, who directed William McIntosh and the Mvskoke warriors to fight the Mvskoke Red Stick faction, provided a firsthand account of these war years. Others who recorded these years included Thomas Woodward and George Stiggins, both of whom fought with Hawkins and McIntosh on the side of the United States. Thomas Woodward, who fought with Andrew Jackson against the Red Sticks, mentioned little about culture, and other than referencing the black drink, he did not mention religion. George Stiggins's father was a Virginia trader, and his mother was Natchez. With regard to religion, he described the preparation and consumption of black drink; the ceremonial smoking of pipes; the activities of the Green Corn festival, including the making of medicine for the ceremony; the spiritual origin of the brass plates, which were sacred objects of Tuckabatchee *tvlwv*; and the ceremonial naming of young men at the Green Corn festival.[15] Stiggins stated that the Green Corn Ceremony "is the only time I ever saw them act as though they paid adoration to the All-Supreme."[16] Stiggins favored acculturation. He wrote:

> In the former days, in the time of the Creeks' . . . undisturbed government, before an agent was located in their nation by the U.S. to improve their morals and reform their customs, their ordained chiefs were more rude, active, despotic, and more frequent in their mandates of tyranny and not nearly so uniform and circumspect in their deportment as now toward the common man.
> All their difficulties in life are caused by their inaction and want of energetic measures.[17]

Not only do these passages reveal Stiggins's sentiments toward traditional Mvskoke ways, but his comments about political methods of the chiefs indicate that he was unfamiliar with many traditional practices. Although his mother was Natchez, Stiggins had been raised in the white world.[18]

The years between the Red Stick War and removal to Indian Territory were desperate ones for the Mvskoke, who attempted to maintain traditional life in the southeastern homeland. Possibly the last description of a Mvskoke religious ceremony in the Southeast is that of John Payne, the author of the song "Home Sweet Home," who witnessed portions of the Green Corn Ceremony at Tuckabatchee *tvlwv* in 1835. He described what he saw in a letter to a relative in New York, along with a lament about the fraudulent means being used in Alabama in 1835 to acquire land from the Mvskoke. Payne appears generally sympathetic to the Mvskoke and is disgusted by the behavior of many of the whites attending the ceremony. Of the Mvskoke he wrote: "I never beheld more intense devotion; and the spirit of the forms was a right and religious one." In contrast to the poor behavior of the whites he encountered at Tuckabatchee in Mvskoke lands, he wrote: "And it was a melancholy reflection for ourselves, that, comparing the majority of the white and red assemblage there, the barbarian should be so infinitely the more civilized and the more interesting of the two." Even though he was sympathetic to the Mvskoke, he reflected that the night dances in the ceremony and the stirring of containers of black drink "reminded me of the witch scenes in Macbeth."[19]

FORCED REMOVAL AND ITS AFTERMATH, 1836–1860
Ethan Allen Hitchcock investigated the fraud involved in providing funds and rations for the Mvskoke during removal and immediately after their arrival in Indian Territory. From 1838 to 1842, he kept journals describing Mvskoke life in their new home. Hitchcock's outrage at the fraudulent treatment is evident in his journals. He was generally sympathetic to the Indians' plight, while viewing them as superstitious and ignorant. He collected some information about religion, including parts of an origin story, medicine practices, encounters with witchcraft, and burial customs.[20] One of the more interesting descriptions he provided was the taking of a drink in 1842 at the new Tuckabatchee *tvlwv* in Indian Territory. The drink sounds like the black drink used so commonly prior to removal. The use of this drink disappeared in Indian Territory due to the difficulty of procuring the leaves of the yaupon, or cassine, from which it was made. Hitchcock's description may be one of the rare accounts of its use in Indian Territory.[21]

Another account of the Mvskoke from the early years in Indian Territory is that of S. W. Woodhouse, a naturalist who left a diary of his adventures for the years 1849 and 1850. This account describes general conditions for the Mvskoke as well as burial practices and the ball game. Other than these comments, his diary includes nothing relating to religion as Woodhouse's interest was in recording information on the flora and fauna of the area.[22]

FIGHTING FOR THEIR LAND ONCE AGAIN:
THE CIVIL WAR TO ALLOTMENT, 1866–1906
G. W. Grayson, the mixed-blood Mvskoke who was active in the fight against allotment and was at one point chief of the tribe, began writing his autobiography in 1908. Shortly thereafter he met John Swanton, the ethnologist who interviewed Jackson Lewis. Grayson became one of Swanton's primary informants. Grayson knew Jackson Lewis well and was present at some of Swanton's interviews with Lewis. In his autobiography Grayson presents a lengthy explanation of his own family history, an invaluable account of the actions of his unit during the Civil War, and an emotional account of the political battles the Nation fought to keep

their sovereignty during the years between the Civil War and allotment. He touches little on the subject of traditional Mvskoke religion. This may be because Grayson was a Christian. He does mention the naming ceremony for male youth and the Indian war medicine some of the men in his regiment used during the Civil War to protect themselves against injury.²³ The maker of that war medicine may have been Jackson Lewis, as Lewis served as an Indian doctor in Grayson's regiment.

During this same difficult period, the Mvskoke employed an attorney, W. O. Tuggle, to represent them in some of their legal claims in Washington. Tuggle spent time with the Mvskoke leaders when they came to Washington and also visited them in Indian Territory. His papers included a diary and sketches written from 1879 to 1882. He was interested in Mvskoke culture and recorded legends and stories. He included a discussion of ball play, the Green Corn Ceremony, and the making of medicine, and he related a medicine song. After observing the making of medicine for a sick child, Tuggle wrote in his diary that he "informed the mother that all this foolishness would do no good." He went on to comment that "the more intelligent [Mvskoke] have left it [the using of traditional medicine] off."²⁴

In 1879 Congress established the Bureau of American Ethnology under the Smithsonian Institution. A primary purpose of this organization was to record the lifeways of the American Indians under the assumption that American Indians would soon disappear due to acculturation and population decimation. The ethnographers of the Bureau of American Ethnology collected and published a significant amount of cultural material from the southeastern tribes during the late nineteenth and early twentieth centuries. The Mvskoke leaders' frequent trips to Washington, D.C. to negotiate with the U.S. government provided ethnographers the opportunity to interview these leaders and learn about the culture without leaving home. The offices of the Bureau of American Ethnology were in Washington, D.C.²⁵

The first of these ethnographers to publish substantial information on the Mvskoke was Albert Gatschet, a Swiss-born linguist educated in Bern and Berlin in philology and theology. His *Migration Legend of the Creek Indians* appeared in 1884. While Gatschet had opportunities to visit the Southeast and Indian Territory, he relied heavily on Mvskoke delegates to the U.S. government who came to Washington, D.C. He made special mention in his work of the following individuals: G. W. Stidham, an unnamed Hitchitee from Eufaula, Chicote, Samuel Checote, Isparhecher, S. B. Callaghan, G. W. Grayson, and David Hodge.²⁶ Gatschet collected and translated migration legends, giving particular attention to Tchikilli's legend. With regard to religion, other than the sacred stories he described as migration legends, Gatschet provided information on belief in spiritual beings like the "holder of breath" and other "genii and mythic animals," and described an initiation into manhood. This initiation description was probably taken from Hawkins's account, as Gatschet mentioned Hawkins and the facts given in both accounts are the same. Gatschet also included a description of the Green Corn Ceremony extracted from Hawkins and Swan.[27]

Another contribution from the ethnographers at the Bureau of American Ethnology was that of J. N. B. Hewitt, who, with J. W. Powell, collected information on the Mvskoke from two Mvskoke leaders in 1881 and 1882.[28] The two leaders were Pleasant Porter and Legus Perryman, both of Okmulgee, Indian Territory. Both were in favor of some acculturation among the Mvskoke and supported the forming of the new constitutional government to replace the traditional system of recognition through towns. Both later served as chief. Porter and Perryman, like Gatschet's informants, were periodically in Washington on Mvskoke business with the federal government, and the taking of these notes during their visits there is likely. With regard to religion, they provided Hewitt with information about the Green Corn Ceremony, medicine people, medicine cures, the soul, the afterlife, and negative use of spiritual forces.

During this period, the Mvskoke who contributed to the written and historical record were preoccupied with the preservation of their nation. Most contributions were in the form of interviews conducted and interpreted by ethnographers, like those already mentioned, or were political commentary or legal transactions authored by the Mvskoke or their representatives. In 1876 the *Indian Journal*, a Mvskoke newspaper, was founded by Indian capitalists under an act of incorporation from the National Council of the Creek Nation. It was one of four papers published in Indian Territory at the time. The paper was organized and run by individuals considered to be in a progressive faction of the Mvskoke. The paper is still published in Eufaula today and is the oldest newspaper in Oklahoma. While this was a Mvskoke paper, in many respects it was like any Euro-American newspaper on the frontier. Rarely were articles published in any language but English. The lifestyle the paper depicted was that of white culture in Indian Territory. The viewpoints presented were in favor of acculturation, although not necessarily in favor of allotment or loss of sovereignty. The most lasting work from the early years of this paper was written by Alexander Posey, who was born near Eufaula in 1873. His mother was Chickasaw and Mvskoke, and his father was white. He grew up in a Mvskoke-speaking household. He favored allotment. His satirical letters to the newspaper signed by the fictitious Fus Fixico were carried in newspapers around the country. Posey wrote the letters in the dialect of a full-blood Mvskoke speaking English and through the letters poked fun at the Dawes Commission.[29] While not focusing on religion, Posey mentions traditional medicine in several of these letters, and one of the characters in these letters is a medicine man. Along with the autobiography of Grayson, who was involved in the production of the *Journal* at one time, the *Journal* provides insight into the views and lives of acculturated, frequently mixed-blood Mvskoke in the years before statehood.

Anthropologists working through the Bureau of American Ethnology continued to add cultural material to the written record. In 1904 and 1905 Frank Speck described medicines and diseases; recorded medicine chants; described religious ceremonies, dances, and dance songs; and discussed origin legends. Most of the information Speck recorded was obtained from Kabitcmaãa (Laslie Cloud) of the Raccoon Clan, a dance leader, ceremonial official, and medicine man of Taskigi *tvlwv* who died in 1905.[30]

STATEHOOD AND LOSS OF
TRIBAL SOVEREIGNTY, 1907–1970

John Swanton, another of the anthropologists employed by the Bureau of American Ethnology, conducted the most comprehensive study yet of Mvskoke culture by a non-Mvskoke. His Mvskoke materials are but a portion of his publishing record; he was a prolific recorder of American Indian life. He visited the Mvskoke in 1910, 1911, and 1912. He worked closely with G. W. Grayson. Zachariah Cook of Wetumka served as his interpreter when Swanton was away from Eufaula, where Grayson lived. Swanton also gained material from Legus Perryman, James Gregory of Okmulgee, and Ellis Childers of Chiaha. As previously mentioned, one of his important informants was Jackson Lewis, and among Swanton's major works on the Mvskoke was *Religious Beliefs and Medical Practices of the Creek Indians.* This two-hundred-page work on Mvskoke religion as well as Swanton's discussions of origin legends and Mvskoke stories found in his other works are a near encyclopedic source on Mvskoke religion as understood by outsiders in the early twentieth century. Topics he discusses include ceremonies like the Green Corn Ceremony, types of medicine people and medicine training, types of medicine, general religious beliefs and deities, and witchcraft and disease. There are many references in appendix B to his specific findings.[31]

While the depression of the 1930s was as devastating in Oklahoma as elsewhere, the decade saw several important contributions to the written record. The most spectacular addition by Mvskoke is in the Indian Pioneer Papers, a project of the Works Progress Administration. The goal of the project was to provide work for the unemployed by collecting from living witnesses vital facts and impressions of pioneer life in Oklahoma. The resulting volumes contain lengthy information on Mvskoke life and history collected in interviews with Mvskoke people. The Indian Pioneer Papers are a rich source of information about Mvskoke history, culture, and daily life from removal through allotment and statehood to the 1930s. There is much information on ceremonies, medicine people, diseases, medicine cures, and religion in general. David Lewis's father, David Lewis, Sr., is one of the interviewees, and interviews include information about both Jackson Lewis and Jeanetta Jacobs, David Lewis, Jr.'s grandmother.[32]

There were several anthropological accounts collected in the 1930s also. John Swanton returned to Oklahoma and the Mvskoke area in the summer of 1929 to gain information about the extant ceremonial grounds. In 1938–39 Mary Haas, a linguist whose major contribution to understanding the Mvskoke is her analysis of Muskogean languages, studied Mvskoke towns in Oklahoma by working with Pa•skó•fa (Johnson Late) of Tuckabatchee, Alex Sulphur of Eufaula, Jasper Bell of Cusseta, and James Hill of Hilabi. Morris Opler, an anthropologist, traveled in the Mvskoke area after the passage of the Oklahoma Indian Welfare Act. In his subsequent report dated 1937, Opler documented the continuing strength of the traditional *tvlwv* and argued that the *tvlwv* should be the unit of organization in any political structure resulting from the Oklahoma Indian Welfare Act. Since his focus was the towns, he did not describe traditional religion. However, he did provide an account of the importance of religion to the Mvskoke, as the towns were frequently focused around religion, either traditional ceremonial grounds or Christian churches. In the course of this work, Opler provided a perceptive description of the interaction between white anthropologists and American Indians. He stated: "Where we [whites] have misconceptions in regard to Indians, we are likely to invite misleading reactions. And since we wanted them and invited them, we are happy to act on a basis of them, frequently moving in the wrong direction."[33]

Alexander Spoehr also conducted anthropological fieldwork among the Oklahoma Mvskoke in the 1930s, specifically in 1938 and 1939, which were the same years Mary Haas was there. Spoehr's focus was the changing kinship patterns among the Mvskoke and the effects of white contact on the same. While he was not studying religion, his work is of interest because, as mentioned earlier, he interviewed Jeanetta Jacobs. His field notes include information gained from talking with her. Others he listed as individuals from whom he gained particularly complete information were Daniel Cook of Lapłako, also interviewed by Haas and the son of one of Swanton's interpreters; Pastor Harjo of Lapłako; Lena Hill, Dick M'Girt, and Jackson Yahoa, all of Tuckabatchee; Willie Sapulpa of Kasihta; Sebin Miller of Tulsa Canadian; and Dan Beaver of Alabama.[34]

INDEPENDENCE REGAINED:
THE MUSCOGEE (CREEK) NATION

In the 1970s, 1980s, and 1990s there was additional recording of Mvskoke religion by outsiders, primarily anthropologists. In 1974 Lester Robbins spent a year participating in the ceremonial cycle of Green Leaf Ceremonial Ground for his work on the persistence of traditional religious practices among the Mvskoke. Toney Hill, the *mekko*, and John Fields, the ceremonial ground *heles-hayv*, were particularly important contributors to his understanding of Mvskoke ceremonials. The 1980 fieldwork of James Howard, an outsider anthropologist, with Willie Lena, chief of Tallahassee Tribal Town, among the Oklahoma Seminoles, resulted in an account of Seminole religion. In this work, Howard is the narrative voice for Lena. The Howard and Lena work is relevant because the Seminoles were members of towns in the Creek Confederacy prior to removal, and after removal the Oklahoma Seminoles maintained or adopted Creek cultural patterns.[35] The Howard and Lena work discusses ceremonies, disease, medicine cures, negative medicine, funeral practices, and spiritual entities, and provides one of the most detailed twentieth-century accounts other than Swanton's. Another relevant work on the Seminoles is Richard Sattler's study of the sociopolitical change in tribal towns from removal to allotment. As a result of his own experiences at the ceremonial grounds, as well as his reading of previous work, Sattler includes discussions of the medicine and the sacred fire. Amelia Rector Bell attended ceremonies at Mvskoke grounds in 1980 and 1981. She recorded information about the ceremonies, medicine, and negative use of medicine, menstrual rules, and types of medicine people.[36]

The Mvskoke themselves have been contributing to this record as well. As a cooperative project with the Oklahoma Indian Affairs Commission, the Thlopthlocco Tribal Town published its own history in 1978. Town members provided the information and prepared the document. Marcellus Williams served as chief data collector and field coordinator, and several elders like Emma Scott, Hettie Burgess, Susie Foster, Jewitt Jimboy, and Sandy Dacon contributed their knowledge. Their publication includes information on the origin of the Mvskoke and of Thlopthlocco *tvlwv*, information on medicine men and their abilities, treatments, and responsibilities, on negative medicine, and on Christianity as well as data on everyday life, food preparation, kinship, and values.[37]

Another written source contributed by a Mvskoke individual was Lewis Oliver's bilingual text of Creek writings published by Bacone College of Muskogee, Oklahoma, in 1985. Bacone is an educational institution in the heart of the Mvskoke area, with the mission of educating American Indian students. Oliver, a member of the Raccoon Clan, was born in 1904. He wrote of the stories of the past, including some references to medicine and to popular Mvskoke stories, like that of the tar baby.[38]

Two published accounts that concern Mvskoke medicine also involve prominent medicine people in David Lewis's family. Marsellus Williams, data collector and field coordinator for the Thlopthlocco Tribal Town history, published a book about his own religious life. He authors this work under the name Bear Heart, an English translation of his Mvskoke name, rather than his English name, Williams. He begins with the training he explains he received from two Mvskoke medicine people, Daniel Beaver and David Lewis, Sr., and continues by examining his experiences with other religious traditions, such as Christianity, the Native American Church, and other American Indian religions.[39]

Chester Scott, full-blood Mvskoke, and Robert Perry, Chickasaw, published a set of stories about the little people, those special entities who appear to medicine people. Perry authored the manuscript, and Scott created the illustrations. The stories are from four generations of Scott's family. The first story told about the little people in their book is the one about Jackson Lewis, which is retold here in chapter 2. Scott explains that, while encounters with the little people are sacred and not to be shared, he is a Christian. "This released him to tell of fun with the 'little people' to the Indian children, and through stories bond child, elder and God." Perry and Scott explain the difference between the Indian and white ways:

> Information about the possibility of native cures touches on the differences of how cultures accept new knowledge. White Man depends on facts and proof, so the limit of believing is as far as his "headlights" reach. The Indian knows that he is one piece of a multi-dimensional world. Indians are observant of the constant change in Nature. Everything in his environment is important. . . . He remembers a lot of information because there was no written language. His memory was uncluttered with unnecessary words and questions. After gathering all the information with his

"headlights," he chooses the "right path" by asking an elder. The elder is the "library." This is the link to the storehouse of knowledge from past generations. . . . An Indian accepts far more on faith alone, which is beyond the known and in the future. This brings peace. . . . The Muscogea People were renown in olden days as the peace-makers.[40]

* * *

Thus for three hundred years, accounts of Mvskoke religion have been appearing in written form. As in any accounting of a colonial history, the accounts reflect the worldviews of their authors as much as the worldviews of their subjects. The accuracy of facts recorded by non-Mvskoke and Mvskoke authors alike is highly dependent on historical time and place and individual perspective. Prior to removal, most contributions are by non-Mvskoke, whose primary interests were in economic and political negotiations with the confederacy. After the removal, the Mvskoke themselves begin to contribute to the written record. The Mvskoke, of course, are not of one mind and their accounts differ according to their personal experiences. Degree of acculturation and religious affiliation are just some of the factors that cause the differences. At the end of the nineteenth century, anthropologists initiated a century of ethnographic work with the Mvskoke, which adds yet another body of work on religion to the record. Like the anthropologist author of this book, authors who are not traditional Mvskoke practitioners of the religion report on that religion with some limitations. They are limited by what Mvskoke practitioners allow them to witness as well as by their own culturally bound abilities to understand a different religious way. This is not to suggest that only Mvskoke practitioners of the traditional religion can provide accurate detail and understanding; rather, it is to emphasize the contextualization of all accounts.

This is the written "setting" into which David Lewis's narrative is placed. What follows in appendix B is a discussion of the specific references in the written record regarding the topics he describes in this book. While demonstrating the continuity of a religious tradition hundreds of years old, these discussions also demonstrate how little is known of Mvskoke medicine in the written tradition. What is captured in print is but a small portion of the complex, living medicine way. Lewis has added to the past written record but has intentionally refrained from committing most of his knowledge to writing. The Mvskoke medicine way continues as a sacred tradition, its fullness found only in oral form.

APPENDIX B

David Lewis's Narrative and the Written Record

CHAPTER 3: KINDS OF MEDICINE PEOPLE

There are no accounts in the written record explaining the types of medicine people as David Lewis explains them. Mentions of medicine people were recorded as early as the eighteenth century. An example of these early comments is from a French naval officer, Bossu, who recounted how he was able to trick a medicine man. His condescension is obvious.

> The Indians have a great deal of confidence in their medicine man, whose hut is covered with skins which he uses for clothing and blankets. He enters the hut completely naked and utters words, understood by no one, in order to invoke the spirit. After that, apparently in a complete trance, he gets up, shouts, and moves about as the sweat pours from every part of his body.
>
> The hut shakes, and the spectators think that this is evidence of the presence of the spirit. The language that the medicine man speaks in his invocations has nothing in common with everyday speech. It is nothing but the product of an overexcited imagination that these charlatans pass off as a divine language. Throughout history, those with a certain amount of ingenuity have been able to fool others.[1]

It is possible that what Bossu was describing was a personal strengthening ritual of a *heles-hayv* in his sweat lodge, as described by Lewis in chapter 4. Whether this is what Bossu witnessed is, of course, not verifiable so many centuries later.

Another early account of medicine people is found in the Hall manuscript of 1775. In this description of encounters with the Mvskoke, Hall mentioned that there was a "Conjuror" in every town who could find lost things, could identify witches, and sometimes was found guilty of witchcraft himself. He stated that the Mvskoke were "very credulous and bigoted to strange traditions."[2] From this account one learns little other than that each town had a *heles-hayv*.

In 1791 Caleb Swan commented on doctors who could be male or female, but were more likely to be female. He described the process of curing: "As all their disorders are to be cured by the herbs and styptics of the woods, assisted by magic, their mode of proceeding is not less singular than superstitious. All physic and decoctions must undergo a process of boiling, stirring, or filtration, attended with blowing, singing, hissing, muttering and a variety of mysterious and sublime operations before it is fitted for use."[3] Thus Swan added to the growing knowledge base the information that a *heles-hayv* could be either male or female and the understanding that curing used plants and religious knowledge. The "blowing" and "singing" he mentioned probably refer to the manner in which the sacred words are put into the medicine using a medicine stick, and indicate the process that is still in use today.

A less condescending and more detailed description of medicine men from the eighteenth century comes from Bartram. In his observations, each town had a medicine man, who had assistants or trainees. He mentioned, as does Hall, that this person could predict the future and perform witchcraft. Bartram explained that the medicine person was much respected and could also cure disease. While he distinguished his view from the one prevailing among Europeans of his day by referring to these medicine people as "priests" rather than "conjurers" and "jugglers," he could not fully accept their powers. He commented that they "pretend" to bring rain and cure disease.

> There is in every town or tribe a high priest, usually called by the white people jugglers, or conjurers, besides several juniors or graduates. But the ancient high priest or seer, presides in spiritual affairs, and is a person of consequence; he maintains and exercises great influence in the state. . . . These people generally believe that their seer has communion with powerful invisible spirits; . . . that he can predict the result of an expedition. . . . and indeed their predictions have surprised many people. They foretell rain or drought, and pretend to bring rain at pleasure, cure diseases, and exercise witchcraft, invoke or expel evil spirits and even assume the power of directing thunder and lightning.[4]

A century later, the descriptions of medicine people usually recognized several types of religious specialists. Hewitt, in the information he collected from Perryman and Porter in Washington in 1881 and 1882, suggested different categories of religious specialists. He identified the "prophet," who could tell the cause of an illness but not cure it. He distinguished the prophet from the medicine person, who could cure. The latter could be male or female. "Sometimes a woman would study medicine and become a doctor but no woman held any office."[5] This medicine person prepared the medicine using herbs or other materials and medicine songs. A town might have multiple medicine people; the "head medicine man of the town" prepared and kindled the council fire. The chief prophet of the town, who could also be a medicine man, prepared the war medicine. Some of the powers of this chief prophet were to "cure or cause fatal illness"; "make the ground quake"; "cause the enemy to lose their way"; "bring rainfall to obliterate tracks"; "lengthen or shorten distances"; "make arrows go straight to the mark"; "transform men into animals such as the wolf or owl"; "cause the warriors to have an aspect terrifying to their enemies"; heal wounds received in war; and "transform the human body into a sieve so as to allow the arrow or bullet to pass through."[6]

Hewitt's use of terms is confusing. *Doctor* and *medicine* man appear to have referred to those who could cure illness. *Prophet* referred to one who could identify diseases but not cure them. In his description of the chief prophet, however, Hewitt stated that this person might or might not be a medicine man, but that the person could cure disease. In Hewitt's understanding, this "chief prophet" also had powers associated with success in war. Regardless of the confusion, Hewitt was identifying at least two categories of religious specialists: prophets who could identify disease and medicine men who could cure disease. How he saw individuals with the other abilities fitting into these two types is difficult to determine.

Speck, in his fieldwork with Laslie Cloud of Taskigi town, uses the term *owalv* to refer to a "shaman," who must first discover the trouble and then make the medicine to cure it.[7] Swanton provided more detail based on his field research in Oklahoma in 1910–12. He used the term *heles-hayv* for the "head priestly functionary" of the ceremonial ground of the town. This individual could be assisted by a number of others, such as medicine mixers, medicine gatherers, and bringers of water for the medicines. This individual might also be the fire builder at the ceremonial ground. In some towns, however, a different individual assumed this role and might be assisted by a wood gatherer. Swanton further distinguished between two other classes of individuals: the knower or prophet called kĕrrv, who diagnosed illness, and the healers called *aliktca* or *heles-hayv*, who were the "repositories of learning," "the guardians of the supernatural mysteries," and the possible possessors of abilities like the ability to fly. Every town had several individuals in this category. Swanton also used the term *doctor* to refer to these *heles-hayv* as well as to those others who knew remedies of a secular nature. He understood that women could be doctors, but assumed that they were "common practitioners" and did not possess sacred knowledge. The doctors who did possess sacred knowledge were also called *isti poskalgi*, fasting men, because their training required them to fast.

Thus Swanton presented several types of religious specialists accompanied by confusing terminology. Probably he meant that there were: (1) doctors who cured using secular remedies; women curers were of this type; (2) *heles-hayv*, also called *isti poskalgi* and *aliktca*, who were repositories of sacred knowledge and cures, and of which a town might have several; they would conduct schools to teach the sacred knowledge and abilities to the young, some specializing in curing specific ailments, like snakebite or war wounds—one did not cure all ailments; (3) a *heles-hayv* who tended to duties at the ceremonial ground, sometimes including building the fire; and (4) *kērrv*, who were the knowers who diagnosed illness.[8] This rendition more closely reflects the explanations of David Lewis, although the carrier/main *heles-hayv* distinction is not made, nor is *owalv* explained.

The distinction between specialists who cure and those who diagnose is well documented, as has already been seen. More support for this distinction is found in written statements from Mvskoke people. In the Indian Pioneer Papers from the 1930s, Nancy Grayson Barnett explained: "There are different kinds of Medicine Men but none will do you any good if you don't have faith in him. . . . There was the herb doctor and the one who blows through a cane into the medicines. Then, there is the prophet or fortune teller who doesn't cure disease."[9] Sandy Fife told a story about the powers of a prophet:

> Talla Massee was an old Indian who died at the age of a hundred and twenty-eight years. He has been dead for four years. He has told us many times of a legend that he couldn't understand at first. When he was a child he heard the old people telling that a prophet had told that some day there would be queer things in the air like ships but not exactly like them. This was foretold before the whites came here. He understood what was meant when he saw the first airplane.[10]

In the 1970s the people of Thlopthlocco Tribal Town recorded information about medicine types that supported the distinction between medicine men and women who cured disease and seers who diagnosed disease. They also supported the data that there could be many medicine people in a town, but only one would have the duties at the ceremonial ground. This individual was required to be of a certain clan.[11]

From her fieldwork in 1980 and 1981, Bell, another anthropologist, explained that she was told that at birth Mvskoke children "know things" and they lose this ability when they begin to speak. They can retain this ability if treated properly. They can as they age become *kērrv*, although Bell knew of only one adult who was.[12] Bell's information differs from that of David Lewis in that she understood that all children at birth had this ability. The others state it is a special gift restricted to a few.

Thus eighteenth-century information provides the knowledge that medicine people were at work in the same medicine-making process still in use in the twenty-first century and that both women and men could be doctors then as now. In the nineteenth-century information, the distinctions between types of religious specialists are suggested, although not clearly explained. In the twentieth century, more detail about these distinctions appears. Both Mvskoke and non-Mvskoke explain that there were prophets and curers and that one male *heles-hayv* of a designated clan served the ceremonial ground. These distinctions are supported by David Lewis, who adds the main *heles-hayv*/carrier distinction. Lewis adds that *owalv*, not *kērrv*, is the proper term to use in referring to a prophet, even though most Mvskoke use *kērrv* to represent prophet. *Kērrv*, on the other hand, is one who "knows" by experience and learning. It is Lewis's intent to correct the written record by adding the main *heles-hayv*/carrier distinction and the *owalv/kērrv* distinction.

CHAPTER 4: THE SELECTION OF MEDICINE PEOPLE
The Selection Process

There is little in the written record about the process of selection of infants. In his work *The Indians of the Southeastern United States*, Swanton states that a child may be raised to be a "wizard" and that twins are particularly "marked out" for such a career.[13] The child raised to be a wizard is kept secluded for the first twenty-four hours of life and fed liquid corn hominy instead of milk. Swanton does not make clear to which southeastern tribe he refers in this passage, although the sources listed as references, Timberlake and Mooney, are describing the Cherokee.[14] Thus one can assume that Swanton is referring to the Cherokee as well. The special nature of twins is mentioned in the Indian Pioneer Papers of the 1930s, which include a comment by Mose Wiley, a Mvskoke of Okchiyae (or Okchayi) Town, who explained that twins "were naturally gifted with the power to foretell and know things."[15]

Just as Lewis explained that the infant is selected for his or her character, there is also some information in the twentieth-century record suggesting that selection was based on aptitude, although the references refer to the selection of youths or adults, rather than infants. Swanton commented that the medicine man for a ceremonial ground was chosen according to fitness rather than descent.[16] Speck, however, explained that for Taskigi *tvlwv*, medicine knowledge was acquired in mythical times.[17] In 1904–5, when Speck gathered his information, medicine knowledge was independently developed, inherited, or purchased. Speck himself purchased medicine songs and formulas from his informant, Kabítcmaãa (Laslie Cloud).

The written record does not contain a description of the infant selection process Lewis describes here. Lewis explains that he thinks the testing and selection process postdates removal and resulted from the actions of medicine people during the removal. As he indicates in the preface, the medicine people were so angry about the removal that they practiced negative medicine against the whites. This turn to the negative by so many medicine people put the entire medicine tradition at risk. Lewis believes that once a medicine person makes bad medicine, he or she can never do only good again. Hence the medicine people called the meeting to decide that in the future, all infants would be tested before being trained. The testing would determine for certain which ones would not be tempted by the negative later in life.

Learning the Plants

There are no other accounts of learning the plants or of a training process like the training Lewis experienced. Early accounts of medicine training among the Mvskoke are sketchy. The first descriptions of these processes date from the late nineteenth and early twentieth centuries and are provided by ethnographers Hewitt and Swanton.[18] Hewitt's information from Perryman and Porter explained the process by which one became a medicine person:

> [A] person must fast a certain number of days, must learn the prescribed songs, must prepare Medicines (and charms) according to well-established formulae, must remain in seclusion at times, and must then use the Medicines which had been thus prepared when called to minister the sick. This process of instruction and initiation continued four moons in each year for four successive years. Each Medicine must be learned in four days.[19]

This brief account gives some sense of the ritual involved in training and the importance of the number four, but does little to explain the training process. Without further detail, it is difficult to determine what type of training Perryman and Porter were describing to Hewitt.

Swanton's work provided more information. He quoted Hawkins's eighteenth-century description of a youth training and suggested that this represented the *posketv* for medicine training, which his own informant described to him.[20] However, Hawkins, who wrote this description in his *Sketch of the Creek Country in the Years 1798, 1799*, entitled it "The Ceremony of Initiating Youth into Manhood."[21] Thus it appears that Hawkins did not intend this description to represent initiation into a medicine society but rather to describe a puberty ceremony. Swanton reinterprets this early ethnographic description as a medicine training rather than the puberty ritual that Hawkins had said it was.[22]

The most complete data on training came from Swanton's own informants and was collected in and around 1910. Swanton attributed much of the detail to Jackson Lewis who described the training process as follows:

> From one to four young men . . . would go into the town and engage some old Indian who was known to have passed through the course and was prepared to teach them. Then all repaired together to a stream of water, usually a densely wooded creek bottom where they were not likely to be observed. . . . The "red root," *miko hoyanidja*, was dug by each candidate, pounded up and put into a pot already provided, and the pot filled with water. Then the instructor came in and blew into the Medicine through a cane. . . . The novice drank great quantities of Medicine . . . so arranging it that by noon he would have taken it four separate times. At noon the instructor came back and then began to tell the novice either by words or songs some of the most elementary things he had to learn. . . . The instructor would tell what to do and what songs to sing in order to give virtue to the Medicine they made for the wounds. . . . Then he instructed him again and said, "Now go over it as I have." He did not stop because his pupil had repeated it correctly once but made him go over it often later, because unless it was gone over in just such a manner it would not be effective when used. . . . The instruction was continued for four successive days. . . . After a month or two, during which the novice went back to the town, he could return to the woods and take another course. . . . Few ever took a complete course. After the fifth or sixth 4-day period one could ask the teacher to put him through the 8-day session, and after that he could ask the teacher to put him through the 12-day session, which was the last. There were very few teachers because very few had passed through the 12-day course. This instruction seems to have required fasting and isolation from noise.

... After the first 4-day session had been gone through a blanket was thrown about the novice and water was poured upon hotter stones inside of this until steam was raised, and after the novice was thoroughly steamed he went to bathe in a cold creek. ... After the education had been completed the old teacher would dig a trench in the ground, put a cane in the novice's mouth so that he might breathe through it, cover him with earth, put leaves over all, and set fire to them. Then he would order the novice to get up and, having done so, he was ready for any emergency in life.[23]

Thus Jackson Lewis provided Swanton with a specific description of a group training process.

David Lewis flatly states that "contrary to modern belief, the Mvskoke medicine people did not have medicine schools for group instruction." Instead, he describes in this chapter a very different process in which Jackson Lewis himself would have been engaged at the time Swanton was interviewing him and collecting the data quoted. The period of the Swanton-Lewis interviews corresponds to the period when Jackson Lewis was training his grandson, David Lewis's father, not as a student in a "medicine school" but as his sole replacement as a main medicine man, in the same process described in chapter 4. Lewis thinks his great grandfather was referring to the training of carriers and that he would not have revealed to Swanton the most sacred training process for his sole replacement as main *heles-hayv*. This may be an example of the way in which the interviewee controls the anthropologist's interview process and the anthropologist's access to information.

More recent twentieth-century accounts of Mvskoke medicine culture are those of Howard and Lena and of Bear Heart and Larkin. Howard and Lena, however, did not comment on the medicine training of a novice. They did comment on adult medicine people learning from each other. Lena mentioned that medicine men might travel a long way to learn a particular formula from another and that sometimes two such individuals would exchange formulas, indicating their respect for each other. He also mentions, however, that formulas might also be jealously guarded and not given out to others.[24] From Lewis's perspective, Lena would have been describing the training of carriers.

Bear Heart, a full-blood Mvskoke, described his own medicine training at length. He recounted the training he received from two well-known medicine men, one of whom was David Lewis, Sr. Bear Heart's account of his training by David Lewis, Sr. differed from the training David Lewis, Sr. gave his own son, David Lewis, Jr. Bear Heart's training occurred while he was an adult and did not include the described initiation. Bear Heart then learned additional religious knowledge from other American Indian cultures, the Native American Church, Christianity, and other religions to form his personal religious beliefs.[25]

Lewis's account of training adds information about a type of training not found in previous accounts. None of these accounts are contradicted by Lewis's assertions, with the exception of Swanton's description attributed to Jackson Lewis. From a distance of ninety years, it is impossible to understand the relationship between Jackson Lewis and John Swanton. Lewis's new information and explanation suggest that the information from Swanton represents a partial understanding.

Initiation

There are few references to medicine initiations in the written record. Adair described an initiation for "Indian priests and prophets," using the "Chickasaw" as an example. This initiation involved a three-day sweat, during which the medicine people could eat nothing but green tobacco and could drink only warm water with button snake root.[26] Swanton commented that he had no evidence beyond what Adair reported of medicine makers and other doctors undergoing a special fast and purification prior to taking their posts. Adair was referring to the Chickasaw tribe. Swanton's reasoning for including the Chickasaw account in his description of Mvskoke religion may have been his belief in the close relationship between the Chickasaw and the Mvskoke. Swanton commented that to the Muskogee tribal towns one might add the Chickasaw, since one band of Chickasaw lived with the Creeks for several years and were held to be of one fire with the Mvskoke town of Cusseta.[27] It remains, however, that Adair's reference does not apply to members of Creek tribal towns of Adair's time but to the Chickasaw. The written descriptions of initiation are thus few and very different from Lewis's. Medicine initiation is one of those aspects of Mvskoke medicine that has simply not been shared with the uninitiated.

Finding the Tunes

Swanton commented on the necessity that songs be learned exactly.[28] He further distinguished between initiates being taught "songs" and "formulas," and described the learning of both. This is different from Lewis's experience, in which the tunes are never learned but must be found by the initiate. Many other recorders of Mvskoke religion commented on the formulas. Speck provided a number of these and, in some cases, the accompanying music.[29] He stated that the words related to the animal causes of the diseases they were used to cure. Howard and Lena recorded several formulas, such as one to cure eagle sickness, one to stop the vomiting of blood, and one to stop bleeding.[30] Lewis refuses to provide any words to the chants he uses, as they are too sacred to be committed to written form. He notes that although Swanton wrote down some of these chants, he learned them from sources other than Jackson Lewis. David Lewis suggests that his great grandfather would not have revealed such sacred information. Lewis is the only one to mention that tunes to the chants were not passed down but that the initiate had to acquire his or her own tunes from the sounds of nature.

Acquiring a Medicine Stick

The medicine stick was mentioned in most accounts of Mvskoke medicine culture. Speck described the "blow-pipe" as a section of cane about thirty inches long that was part of the Creek medicine paraphernalia and stated that it is not preserved with any particular reverence.[31] Swanton suggested that the cane and plants could be provided by the family for whom the medicine person was making medicine.[32] Howard and Lena referred to the stick as a "bubbling tube" and described its use as a way to mix the "tea" of a medicine that is steeped or boiled.[33] Howard understood that it added strength to the medicine. He described the tube as a "two-foot length of hollow native cane" that was considered a sacred instrument. Lewis affirms Howard's understanding of the sacred nature of the medicine stick. Contrary to Swanton's assertion, Lewis states that in his experience, the stick is never provided by the patient. Lewis's experience is that the cane can be of any length. Its sacred preparation is essential, but its length is a matter of convenience.

There are several accounts of the use of medicine sticks by Mvskoke tribal members. Alexander Posey, the well-known early twentieth-century Mvskoke poet, journalist, and newspaper editor, described the use of the medicine stick in one of the satirical letters he wrote under the fictional identity of Fus Fixico.[34]

> Old Choela was sure good doctor. He was just take his grubbing hoe and go out in the woods and dig up lots medicine anywhere. Then he was take his cane and blow in the medicine pot long time and sing little song with it, too, like at busk ground. But he aint want no monkey business round there neither while he was fixing that medicine. . . . The medicine what Choela was give you taste good all right too, you bet. Taint stink like white man medicine.[35]

Other mentions of the medicine stick can be found in the Indian Pioneer Papers. The following is an example:

> When one felt stiff in his joints, a squaw would take her children to the woods, by a small branch, and gather herbs to brew. She would take the bark from a cottonwood tree and boil it in spring water. Then she would take a hollow reed about thirty inches long and blow in the liquid. This she would do for four mornings. All the time she was blowing in the liquid she faced the east. . . . While preparing this medicine, the squaw would drink "sofky," a drink made from corn similar to hominy. She felt that would teach her a medicine song for the particular disease she was preparing the medicine for.[36]

Thus the use of the stick is well documented, but its sacred nature and sacred preparation as described by Lewis have not been described previously in the written record.

Help from Teachers

Spiritual help during dreams is recorded elsewhere. Hewitt was told that girls could acquire guardian spirits through dreams and that youths, when fasting at the time of puberty, might be visited by *Innutska* ("what comes to him in sleep").[37] Swanton cited Adair's comments on the Chickasaw, who told of being in communication with "holy spirits or angels."[38] This was, again, a reference to the Chickasaw and not directly to the towns of the Creek Confederacy of which Adair had knowledge. Swanton wrote that at the time of his fieldwork, "even in the cases of the graduates [medicine doctors] the power acquired through their training no longer appears to be associated with supernatural guardian spirits. Such, however, was evidently the case in former days." He further commented, however, that a fear of ghosts did continue to exist. Thus nothing as specific as Lewis's description of the role of deceased medicine people as helpers is found in the record.

To sum up: There are scattered written references to selection and training of medicine people. Found in the previous record are references to marked religious ability in some infants, the dependence of selection on the individual's aptitude, training of adults in medicine schools and individually, the learning of medicine songs, the use of medicine sticks, and the communication with guardian spirits during dreams. The training process for a main *heles-hayv* is more complicated than previously indicated. It is Lewis's interpretation that the previous reports of Swanton and others must have referred to the training of carriers rather than main *heles-hayv*. By contrast, the training of a main *heles-hayv* begins at birth and is accompanied throughout by the taking of medicine. The training is complete by approximately the age of ten. David Lewis's description of this process suggests that the uninitiated, and especially the non-Mvskoke, have little understood the depth and intensity of this sacred training. Previous written accounts do not describe the selection, training, testing, and initiation of a child as a sole replacement for a main *heles-hayv*. They do not include the sacred preparation of the medicine stick or the ceremonial passing of a medicine stick from teacher to young initiate. They do not explain that when sacred medicine formulas are taught, only the words are passed on and not the tunes, as the tunes are unique to each individual. Nor do they describe the role of deceased medicine people in the lives of the living, in that living *heles-hayv* can be aided by the old ones through dreams and visions.

Further, not all the towns in the Creek Confederacy before removal or in the Oklahoma Mvskoke Creek tribe after removal spoke the same Muskogean language, and some did not speak Muskogean languages at all; both Lewis's teachers were from towns and clans that did speak Muskogean languages. Lewis's grandmother and father were probably trained by individuals from different tribal towns and clans who spoke different Muskogean languages (Jackson Lewis was Hitchitee). However, they taught him the same sacred story, the same uses for plants, and the same preparation of medicine sticks, and they conducted the same type of initiation. Only the words to the chants and the words used during initiation were different. Thus there may have been some unity in the manner in which Mvskoke medicine was practiced in the twentieth century, even though the members of the *tvlwv* of the confederacy spoke nine languages.

CHAPTER 5: MEMORIES OF CHILDHOOD IN A MEDICINE FAMILY

Memories of childhood are found in many twentieth-century accounts by Mvskoke.[39] Some of these contain memories of relatives who were medicine people. This recollection found in the Indian Pioneer Papers is from Summa Buckner:

> I am the great grandnephew of the early leader and spokesman of what was the early Ochai tribe. He was called and known as Ho-tul-kee E-math-la. He was the man that led the Ochai tribe to what was the new country to be their home. I have seen him, been with him and have actually heard him tell of many things he had

seen and of the many things he had done. . . .

Many of his words seemed to prophesy and although I was small then I later realized some of the things that he had spoken were coming true. . . .

He said, "In days to come you will see the making of things running across the country having the appearance of ribs." This he referred to the railroads. "Other things will be placed in the air and be like the spider's web." This was the telegraph and telephone wires.

One late evening just as the sun was setting in the west, he asked me if I could see the red streak and path made by the sun in its course during the day. He moved his hand from the East to the West in an arched fashion yet I had to answer him that I could not see what he was able to see.[40]

The little people, whom Lewis discusses in this chapter, were previously mentioned in chapter 2, as both Lewis's great grandfather, Jackson Lewis, and his father, David Lewis, Sr., knew them as well. There are other accounts of the little people in the written record. Tuggle collected stories about them in the 1880s, and Swanton wrote about a story he heard from a Natchez man.[41] In the story Swanton retold, the man's father was hunting and had no luck. He encountered little people wearing caps and carrying bows and arrows. They led him to a place where he found medicine in a little stone cup. He drank it and later killed a deer.[42] The little people are known to make those who encounter them confused, thus bringing trouble rather than help. They are most likely to appear in a helpful guise to medicine people and to children. Howard and Lena wrote that Wesley Green, a Seminole, had a grandson who often played with the little people.[43] They can tell future events. In one story Howard heard, a child saw the little people moving out of their house and putting all their belongings in tiny wagons because their house was to be destroyed. Later a tornado did destroy the trees they lived in.

Mvskoke people have written and spoken about them also. Oliver recounts encounters with the little people and, of course, Perry and Scott have written a book of little people stories, including the one about Jackson Lewis quoted in chapter 2.[44] There are several accounts of them in the Indian Pioneer Papers. Mose Lasley explained that "the little people make their homes in the trees of the woods and those homes can be distinguished by the extra thick growth with small twigs of branches in the trees, but the homes cannot be found in every tree. . . . They take the very large objects as being very small and cannot do the small work while a small work is large to them."[45] Willia Roberts explained that the little people use raccoons to hunt with, as humans would use dogs, and if a person was not bewitched by them, the person did not have the power to see them.[46]

Lewis's recollections in this chapter add to the previous record collected in the twentieth century about the activities of medicine people and also of the little people.

CHAPTER 6: THE STORY

In this chapter, Lewis tells parts of the sacred story about the origin of medicine plants. Other accounts of the origin of medicines appear in early versions of a Creek migration legend. Possibly the earliest known version of a migration legend including references to plants was the one Tchikilli delivered to Governor Oglethorpe in 1735 at Savannah, a portion of which is quoted in chapter 1.[47] Gatschet and Swanton, two of the first ethnographers to work with the Mvskoke materials, both reviewed migration legends a century and a half after Tchikilli narrated this one to Oglethorpe.[48] Swanton suggested that Tchikilli (or Chekilli) was probably a Cusseta and attributed the legend to Cusseta sources. Tchikilli was referred to as "emperor of the Upper and Lower Creeks," although it is clear there would not have been a single leader of the Creeks in the early eighteenth century. The legend Tchikilli related explained that during their migration to their homeland, four plants revealed themselves to the people and explained their uses. These were the medicine plants: *pasaw* (*passv*), rattlesnake root; *micoweanochaw* (*mēkko-hoyvnēcv*), red root; *sowatchko*, which grows like wild fennel; and *eschalapootchke*, little tobacco.[49]

Hawkins, the U.S. agent to the Mvskoke prior to removal, recounted a migration legend he learned from Taskaya Miko of Appata-I, a branch village of Cusseta in 1798. The legend included reference to acquiring four medicines. Thus the legend Hawkins related and that of Tchikilli would both be from Cusseta *tvlwv*. In the Hawkins version, four visitors from four corners of the world came to the people. Each of the four showed them plants. Some plants were not recollected, for a total of seven plants were revealed. The plants Hawkins identified are *micco hoyonejau* (*mēkko-hoyvnēcv*, red root), *anchenau* (*vcenv*, cedar), *passau* (*passv*, button snake root), and *too loh* (sweet bay).[50] Bartram, traveling the Mvskoke lands from 1773 to 1776, provided an account of this Creek legend that coincided closely with the versions by Tchikilli in 1735 and Taskaya Miko in 1798.[51] Thus these three eighteenth-century non-Mvskoke chroniclers described similar legends, which can be traced to Cusseta *tvlwv* and its branch villages.

In the nineteenth century, Hitchcock, attorney for the Mvskoke shortly after removal, learned scattered pieces of an origin story at the new Tuckabatchee *tvlwv* in Indian Territory in 1842.[52] His version includes a reference to the origins of tobacco and corn. In this story a woman died and was buried by the side of a large hill, and from her grave a stalk of corn sprang up. Tobacco grew from the rib of a woman under the same circumstances. Hitchcock also was told a story in which God sent a man to make the earth, and after he had made it, God said to the Indian, "Here is wood, cedar and poplar . . . , for you to use." Hitchcock's legends from the postremoval period are different from the legends collected prior to removal from Cusseta *tvlwv*.

In the twentieth century, again only pieces of legends are recorded. Swanton mentioned the legend presented by Tchikilli and the accounts of Hawkins and Gatschet. In describing the legends explaining the origin of the *boskita* (or *posketv*, the Green Corn Ceremony), Swanton stated that "the Creeks of the present day [1910–12] for the most part know only that it was established in the beginnings of things for the benefit of the Indians."[53] He cited Big Jack of Hilibi, who told him that *Ifofanga* (*epohfvnkv*, The One Above) gave the Indians the *passv* (button snake root) and *mēkko-hoyvnēcv* (red root) to keep as long as time should last. Sanger Beaver, a Tcatoksofka (Cvtaksofkv), told Swanton that in ancient times people were continually fighting, and one man fasted on the trouble and finally was given *mēkko-hoyvnēcv*, *passv*, and some other medicines, along with songs for each. The fasting man said this was "for the building up of our future generations, to make grow up the women and children." He then started the fire of the confederacy, and other Indian tribes came there and obtained their fires from that fire. Swanton's informant knew there was much more to the story, but he did not know it.

Swanton also related several versions of a legend acquired from members of Tuckabatchee *tvlwv*.[54] One version Swanton recorded from town member Alindja, with George W. Grayson serving as translator. Alindja's account describes a meeting of representatives from the towns of Coweta and Tuckabatchee, during which they exchanged medicines. The Tuckabatchee medicine was *mēkko-hoyvnēcv* and the Coweta medicine was *kvpvpaskv* (spicewood). In another of the versions, the Coweta medicine was *passv* (button snake root). Subsequent to the encounter, the Tuckabatchee and Coweta used both medicines. Swanton was told that the last person to know the origin myth in its completeness was Napoleon Yahola, who died before the Civil War. Speck, collecting data in 1904 and 1905, states that in the origin myth of Taskigi *tvlwv*, various animals and creatures in the mythical age arbitrarily introduced disease and agreed to make cures consisting of song formulas and medicines.[55]

Thus there are several references to legends about the origin of the medicine plants in the written record. Given the variation in tribes that made up the Mvskoke Confederacy, the autonomy of towns, and the individual knowledge of medicine people prior to removal and into the twentieth century, it is possible that there were different stories about the origin of medicine. It is likely as well that the Mvskoke did not wish to share these sacred stories with outsiders. In this book Lewis also is sharing only a fragment of the sacred story told by his family. He comments that he learned the same origin story from his maternal grandmother and from his father. This experience suggests the possibility that there has been some degree of unity among the twentieth-century Mvskoke regarding religious knowledge. The historical data are limited and the medicine heritages of the storytellers in the record are unknown. There could have been great variation among medicine people since each initiated *heles-hayv* was passing along a tradition shared only by a single individual to whom it was taught. In addition to that, the numerous clans, the independence of the *tvlwv*, and the changes through the centuries could account for many differences.

CHAPTER 7: PLANTS

David Lewis chose to comment on plants from Swanton's published plant list.[56] Thus Swanton's list includes references to all the plants Lewis describes. Another important plant list is provided in Howard and Lena.[57] References to the plants Lewis discusses are given below.

1. Mēkko-hoyvnēcv (Salix humilis)

Lewis translates the Mvskoke name as "King passing through," and the story of the origin of this medicine and the reason for its name is told in chapter 6. This plant is referenced extensively in the written record as one of the important medicine plants. The first mention of it occurs in Tchikilli's origin legend presented in 1735. Swanton translates the name as "passer by of the chiefs," which is a similar translation to Lewis's.[58] As described in chapter 1, the word *mēkko* traditionally referred to the leader of a tribal town and could be translated into English as either "chief" or "king." From George Grayson, Swanton learned that this medicine was "supposed to pass by of its own power."

From her fieldwork in the 1980s, Bell translates this name as "wild chief."[59] The use of this translation for the name is mentioned by Chilli Barnett of the Alabama tribe in an interview from the 1930s. Barnett explained:

This particular herb now known as the "Wild King" did not always have that name. It was called by several different names but was eventually named after an old Alabama chief.

As the story is told, there was a man whose name was Ko-hag-a-me, a chief once of the Alabama tribe. Some of the older Alabama Indians have told and the story has been handed down that during the time that Ko-hag-a-me was leader and chief of the tribe, and in the time of battle or trouble, this chief would urge his warriors into the battle and sneak away and hide out every time so that he was nicknamed the "Wild King."

The herb mentioned was used by the Alabama tribe of Indians during the days of Ko-hag-a-me and that herb received the name of "Wild King" and has been known by that name ever since.[60]

The differences between the Alabama story and translation of Wild King and Lewis's story and translation may be due to different traditions in different towns.

As Lewis states, this plant is used for many sicknesses. Some specific sicknesses are found in the written record. Swanton lists the following: fever with nausea and vomiting (information from Jackson Lewis); fever, malaria, and biliousness (information from Caley Proctor); for dropsy, headache, and the curing of deer sickness (from unidentified sources); and as one of the plants used in curing of "blood of the bear" sickness (in which the patient spits up blood continually). Swanton also states that it was used with spicewood (*kvpvpaskv*) to bathe in for rheumatism and swelling. In combination with *passv*, it could be used to cure "the clap." In conjunction with other ingredients, it was a cure for "sun disease," which gave the patient a sensation of heat in the crown of the head, produced general aches, and caused him to become lightheaded and to collapse around midday. It was also involved in a cure for the sickness a man could get when exposed to a woman during her menstrual period and for problems caused by the ghost of a dead person.[61] Speck reports use of this medicine to cure headaches caused by the deer.[62] This may refer to the same use Swanton calls a cure for deer sickness. Tuggle lists it as used in cures for headaches.[63] There are several references to red root in the interviews conducted in the 1930s for the Indian Pioneer History Project. For example, Nancy Grayson Barnett stated, "It is good for most everything. To get rid of the poisons of the body, like when you ache all over, or have fevers or want to eat green corn."[64]

The plant is reportedly used in ways that do not involve the curing of sickness. Many written accounts of the *posketv*, the Green Corn Ceremony, describe the use of this plant in that annual ceremony just as Lewis does.[65] A good review of written references regarding this is found in Howard, who specifically stresses the importance of *mēkko-hoyvnēcv* in the Green Corn Ceremony.[66] In that ceremony, the participants bathe with medicine made with this plant and also drink medicine made with it. After drinking it, they vomit. Howard states that the plant itself is not an emetic; in his opinion, the vomiting is a cultural rather than a biological act. Jefferson Berryhill, interviewed in the 1930s, also described use of red root.

> Early in the morning before the sun is up a person or an Indian is up. He fixes the medicine by putting the scraped bark in the jar or bucket of water then takes a small arrow size bamboo he blows in the water and chants some kind of magic. He sings of things that no man can understand unless he was gifted to learn. After some length of time after he had made his medicine he gets up. Faces the rising sun and begins to drink the medicine. He keeps drinking it till he gets so full he begins to vomit, he vomits till he is weak or till he has vomit all the films out of his lungs then he washes his face with the medicine, also his hands. Then he eats his breakfast. This is repeated four times in succession. This is done at the change of the moon, when it's new moon. The Indians were healthy long ago by living up to their customs.[67]

In Berryhill's account, a logical assumption is that this was a purification measure by a medicine person. Thus there is information in the written record about two of the five uses of *mēkko-hoyvnēcv* that Lewis provides. Those two are the curing of sicknesses and the use at the ceremonial ground. The other three (doctoring a house, cleaning witchcraft out of a person, and relieving stress) are new references. In all these uses, the plant is the same, but the chants differ according to the use. The record on *mēkko-hoyvnēcv* supports Lewis's statement that this was one of the main medicine plants.

2. *Passv (Eryngium yuccifolium)*
This plant, also known as button snake root, is likewise well documented in the written record. Jackson Lewis stated that its primary use was in curing snakebite and that is was also used in conjunction with the "deer potato" for rheumatism, known as "deer disease." In addition, it could be used in a cure for catarrh, a disease associated with a grub that lives in the nostrils of deer.[68] David Lewis provided additional information in describing how the medicine is applied when used for rheumatism. Howard

and Lena again provide a review of much of the written record. As David Lewis states, a medicine made with this plant is important in the Green Corn Ceremony. Howard and Lena describe in detail the method of taking the medicine internally using two fingers and offering to the four directions.[69] Lewis's other description of use at the beginning of the Green Corn Ceremony, when a needle or thorn is dipped in a medicine made with this root and then the recipient is scratched with the sharp implement, is not found in other sources. References to the scratching ceremony are common in descriptions of the Green Corn Ceremony, but references to the use of *passv* in the medicine in which the thorn is dipped are not common.

The earliest mention of *passv* is found in Tchikilli's origin story in 1735. He described the finding of four medicines. Like *mēkko-hoyvnēcv*, *passv* was one of the four. These medicines spoke to the people explaining their uses. Caleb Swan and Benjamin Hawkins, observing Mvskoke culture in the 1790s, both mention the use of *passv* in a medicine used in war.[70] Hawkins further mentions it being used by young men undergoing initiation into manhood. That initiation ceremony description by Hawkins is the one Swanton later labels as an initiation for medicine men. Swanton provides other uses for *passv* besides the ones he specifically references to Jackson Lewis. From Caley Proctor he learned that it could be used for neuralgia and for kidney problems, from Zachariah Cook that it could be used for diseases of the spleen, and from an unidentified source that it was used to cleanse the system and purify the blood.[71] In addition to its use in the medicine in which the thorn for scratching at ceremonies is dipped, uses David Lewis mentions that have not been previously recorded are for treating worms in children, and for venereal disease and high fever. Like *mēkko-hoyvnēcv*, however, *passv* is an important medicine referenced in the earliest accounts from the eighteenth century and still of importance at the beginning of the twenty-first century.

3. Heles-Hvtke (Panax quinquefolium)
Known as ginseng in English, this is another important medicine plant. David Lewis's description of it as used in medicine to cure shortness of breath was mentioned by Caley Proctor and Jackson Lewis in Swanton's work and by Homer Emarthle and Willie Lena in Howard's work. Swanton also explained that it could be used in medicines to treat croup in children (learned from Jackson Lewis), coughs so severe that they cause a patient to become hoarse (Swanton states this is called the "millepede" disease), and fevers with which the patient cannot sweat. In line with these treatments for cough, Susie Ross Martin, interviewed for the Indian Pioneer Project,

explained that it was used for pneumonia, which was called "winter fever." Proctor and Lewis both told Swanton it could be used to stop bleeding from a cut. Proctor provided Swanton with the formulas he knew to be used with *heles-hvtke* in stopping blood and shortness of breath, respectively. Also, Swanton explains, it can be used to keep away ghosts. Lena informed Howard that the plant could be used in medicine that a man could use to attract a woman or in medicine to cure a nosebleed. David Lewis mentions its use for shortness of breath, and his mention of its use for protection may correspond to Swanton's understanding that it is used to keep away ghosts. The other uses described by Lewis are not found in these other sources.[72]

4. Notossv (*Angelica atropurpurea*)

Swanton was told by Jackson Lewis that this plant was used in medicine to cure back pains in adults and as a vermifuge for children. David Lewis concurs with these uses. The earliest mention of this plant is by Bartram in his travels as a naturalist in the Creek area from 1773 to 1776. He comments that it was used in medicines to relieve problems of the stomach and intestines and for colic and hysterics. Two hundred years later, Willie Lena told Howard the plant is still in use for curing hysterics. A cloth soaked in an infusion of the medicine was placed on the ailing person's forehead. Other than the uses described by his great grandfather, David Lewis explains that, like two hundred years ago, the plant is still used for stomach disorders. The other uses he mentions—preventing heat stroke during the Ribbon Dance in the Green Corn Ceremony, aiding ceremonial singers, and curing legal problems are uses not present in the record.[73]

5. Welanv (*Chenopodium ambrosioides*)

Jackson Lewis's only comment on the plant known in English as wormseed was that it was used in curing many ailments. The earliest mention of this plant is from Hawkins, who in the eighteenth century listed it as one of the fourteen medicines used in the Green Corn Ceremony. Usage in this ceremony is still occurring today. Other than David Lewis's reference to it, Swanton and Howard both describe its use at Green Corn ceremonies in the twentieth century. Like *mēkko-hoyvnēcv* and *passv*, there is documentation that this plant has been used in the Green Corn Ceremony for at least two hundred years. Caley Proctor told Swanton the plant was used to cure fever, a use David Lewis also mentions, and Howard, like Lewis, mentions its use in curing worms in children. David Lewis's mention of the use of *welanv* to cure sore eyes is not recorded in these other sources.[74]

6. Vcenv

Swanton learned from Jackson Lewis that sprigs of cedar could be applied warm to areas where the patient felt pains or aches and from Caley Proctor that it was used in a tonic to thin the blood. Jackson Lewis mentions it as one of the ingredients in a medicine for "deer disease," which has the symptoms of rheumatism, and in "good-snake disease."[75] Swanton says William McCombs explained that "eagle disease," manifested by cramps in the neck muscles, could be cured with cedar fumes. Swanton lists it as one of the plants used in "gathering on land" disease caused by the little people and giants. Cedar is used in this cure because giants fed on the berries of the cedar. Cedar is also mentioned by interviewees in the 1930s in the Indian Pioneer Project. Bun Ryal, for example, mentions that cedar was burned and the smoke inhaled for colds and fever.[76] David Lewis confirms usage in the manner Jackson Lewis described, but does not mention the use as a blood thinner. David Lewis additionally comments on its usage with other plants for many ailments and its use in smoking out homes.

7. Kvpvpaskv (Lindera benzoin)

The English name for this plant is spicewood or spicebush. Hawkins mentions it as one of the fourteen medicines used in the Green Corn Ceremony in the 1790s.[77] Lena confirms that the plant was still used in the Green Corn Ceremony by the Oklahoma Seminoles in 1980.[78] In the twentieth century, Swanton states that it was used in water either by taking it internally or by steaming the body in the liquid in order to reduce pains and aches. It was used along with mēkko-hoyvnēcv to produce vomiting and purify the blood and, in another cure, used with mēkko-hoyvnēcv to cure pains caused by association with a grave. It was in addition used along with other plants in a cure for those afflicted by the spirit of war. Swanton mentions no reference to this plant from Jackson Lewis.[79] Reasons for lack of mention could be many. Perhaps Swanton did not ask him about this plant. In the first use David Lewis mentions, kvpvpaskv can be used as a substitute for mēkko-hoyvnēcv as a purification at funerals. This is similar to Swanton's reference. Lewis's other uses may be additions to the record.

8. Kofockv-rakko (Monarda sp.)

Called horsemint, Swanton states that Mvskoke use this plant to induce perspiration and to cure delirium. It was used in a cure for "gathered on land" disease caused by the little people and the giants and in a cure for a disease caused by the spirit of war. For both diseases, the symptoms could be delirium. Caley Proctor explained it was combined with *mēkko-hoyvnēcv* to cure dropsy and swelling in the legs. Howard and Lena state that it was often mixed with other medicines to make them taste good. Nancy Grayson Barnett mentions that it was put on the tonsils from the inside. Swanton does not mention any uses given by Jackson Lewis. Proctor's reference to its use in curing swelling in the legs probably corresponds to David Lewis's reference to its use by shell shakers for swelling in the feet and legs. The other uses Lewis provides are not mentioned in these sources.[80]

9. Kvtohwv

Other than Lewis's explained uses, Swanton states that honey locust was used to prevent disease, not to cure it. The sprigs, thorns, and some branches are chopped and boiled in water. The users bathe in this to prevent themselves from catching diseases like smallpox and measles. It is used for four days in a row. Lewis comments that this plant can be used to stupefy fish. Several plants could be used to stupefy fish, the best known and best documented being *haloneske*, or devil's shoestring, which Lewis also mentions.[81]

10. Vlv (Aesculus sp.)

This plant, also known as buckeye, was a strong medicine used in small quantities, according to Swanton. The roots are used for pulmonary consumption and can be used for this in conjunction with haloneske or devil's shoestring. *Vlv* can also be used to stupefy fish. Swanton does not attribute this information to any specific informants and does not mention any information on this plant provided by Jackson Lewis.[82] Jefferson Berryhill, interviewed for the Indian Pioneer Project, also mentions the use of buckeye to kill fish, explaining that devil's shoestring was preferable because buckeye was so strong that it did not give the fish a "sporting chance."[83] David Lewis adds the use of *vlv* for cataracts, unrecorded previously, and the carrying of a seed for good luck.

11. Haloneske or Aloneske (Tephrosia virginiana)

This is devil's shoestring, the most important of the plants used by tribes of the Southeast to stupefy fish so that they could be easily caught. This usage is mentioned several times by individuals interviewed for the Indian Pioneer Project.[84] Jackson Lewis told Swanton this plant was used in medicine to treat pulmonary consumption. Other uses Swanton lists are Zachariah Cook's explanation that the plant is used with *wēso* (sassafras) in treating "perch sickness," a disease in which the patient has severe bouts of coughing. It can also be used for "turtle sickness," manifested as chronic cough. Caley Proctor explained that it was used to treat bladder problems, impotence, and irregular menstrual periods.[85] David Lewis refers to the use of this plant in stupefying fish and for treating bladder problems, as described previously in the written record. He adds an explanation of its use for treating varicose veins and gun-shot wounds.

12. Vtakrv-lvste (Baptisia sp.)

The Mvskoke term translates as "black weed." The use David Lewis describes is unrecorded in the other written sources. Swanton lists a single use: to treat children who are drowsy and lifeless and about to get sick. Alec Berryhill in the Indian Pioneer Papers mentions that the roots were used but does not explain what they were used for.[86]

13. Cvto-heleswv

This translates as "rock medicine," and Swanton describes it as grow-ing in clumps with a blue flower in early spring. He states that it is used only when the old medicine men are making the novices fast. Swanton was referring to the plant called cvto-heleswv.[87] Thus David Lewis adds the explanations of the use of the plant and of the use of the rock to the written record.

14. Yvnvsv-heleswv

The previously recorded use for this "bison medicine" is Swanton's record-ing that this medicine was placed on the tongue of a newborn child and this would make the child strong, robust and daring.[88] This corresponds to David Lewis's usage of it in a bath to make children strong and husky.

15. 'To-heleko (Phoradendron sp.)

The leaves and branches of mistletoe were reported by Swanton to be used as one of the ingredients in medicine to treat consumption and other lung trouble. Swanton's references to the use of this plant are confusing. He states that it is one of the ingredients in the medicine used to cure an ailment caused by the little people, which is called "gathered on land" or "outside gathering on land" and occurs when the little people cause persons to become bewildered and led astray. 'To-heleko is used in conjunction with Pvkanvho, vcenv, coskv, pvrko-rakko, and several other plants in a medicine to treat this ailment. Swanton then states that Zachariah Cook told him this disease was pneumonia and hece-pakpvkē was in the medicine.[89] Speck, from his fieldwork conducted at about the same time, reports use of 'to-heleko in medicine to cure a sickness caused by the raccoon, in which the patient experiences sleeplessness and sadness. The first two uses David Lewis lists correspond to the ones given by Swanton and Speck. David Lewis's final use, for the little people to use themselves, is a different usage concerning the little people than the one Swanton provides.

16. Akhatkv (Platanus occidentalis)
In Mvskoke this translates as "white down in," according to Swanton, and it is known to English speakers as sycamore. Chips from the tree and bark were used in a medicine for treating pulmonary tuberculosis, and in combination with *akcelvlaskv* and *akwahnv*, this is used in treating "gathers in the waters" disease, an ailment in which one vomits and has pain in the stomach and bowels. In combination with *akcelvlaskv, akwahnv,* and *vcenv,* it is used to cure "good-snake disease," according to Jackson Lewis.[90] None of the uses David Lewis describes are found in these other accounts.

17. Akcelvlaskv (Betula sp.)
Known to English speakers as white birch, Swanton states this was used in medicine for pulmonary tuberculosis.[91] The uses David Lewis describes are not recorded for the Mvskoke.

18. Akwahnv
A previously recorded use for this is Swanton's explanation that families used willow in the summer to prevent fever by boiling the roots and bathing in and drinking the resulting liquid. Swanton also records it as a plant used in "gathers in the waters" disease, which causes stomach pains and vomiting. Jackson Lewis told him it was an ingredient in "good-snake disease."[92]

19. Coskv (Quercus stellata)
This plant is known to English speakers as post oak. Other references to its use include one from Jackson Lewis, who told Swanton that the bark was used to make a drink to treat dysentery. Swanton also describes its use in conjunction with other plants in a medicine for "spirit of war" disease, an ailment in which a person who is not otherwise ill talks deliriously about war, and in "gathered on land" disease.[93] Lewis's use of this for ridding the patient of sores is not found in the other accounts.

20. Pvkanvho (Prunus sp.)
A previous reference to uses of this plant among the Mvskoke is Swanton's statement that the roots are boiled and used in a medicine for dysentery. Swanton mentions it as one of the ingredients in the medicine for "gathered on land" disease.[94] Lewis's three uses are not included in these.

21. Tvfosho (Ulmus sp.)

Elm is used for toothache, according to Jackson Lewis. Swanton states that Jackson Lewis "thought that the branches were taken, but there was a secret about its use which the doctors who knew about it did not divulge and he was not acquainted with it." David Lewis explains that in curing toothache with *tvfosho* the inner bark is used but not the branches, and explains how this is prepared. Susie Ross Martin told the interviewer for the Indian Pioneer Project that the bark was used as a poultice to reduce inflammation and that the water from it was used as a drink for fevers.[95]

22. Pvrko-rakko (Vitis palmata)

This is called "big grape." Swanton explains that this was used for tonsillitis and as a substitute medicine for snakebite when the preferred plant was not available. Swanton also lists it as another of those ingredients in medicine for "gathered on land" disease. Howard and Lena report that it was used for diabetes, cavity prevention in children, and to promote hair growth or prevent baldness. They also report the same usage David Lewis reports, to secure the return of a wandering spouse.[96]

23. Tartahkv (Populus deltoides)

This is known in English as cottonwood. Swanton reports the same usage for repairing broken bones that David Lewis reports.[97]

24. Wēso (Sassafras sp.)

Swanton reports that *wēso* was used in a medicine for "dog disease," the symptoms of which were severe pain in the bowels and stomach and vomiting. Swanton also mentions *wēso* as an ingredient in the cure for "thunder disease," which causes severe pain in the arms and head and in "perch disease," acute coughing. Howard and Lena report its use for chest pains. Tuggle explained its use in curing rheumatism or dropsy caused by association with a grave.[98] The uses Lewis describes do not appear in these sources.

25. Hece-pakpvke (Lobelia sp.)

Swanton suggests that this is a species of *Lobelia*. The name translates as "tobacco bloom." David Lewis agrees with the comment Swanton attributes to Jackson Lewis, namely, that this plant was difficult to find and highly valued, was older than smoking tobacco, and was with the Creeks "from the beginning." Willie Lena suggests the same. Tuggle provides an origin story for this medicine. It was used in many kinds of cures and was used to ward off ghosts. Zachariah Cook said it was used for a disease he called pneumonia, and Swanton states it was used for "gathered on land" disease caused by the little people and giants.[99]

26. *Poyvfekcv-heleswv*

David Lewis says this is not a plant but rather a problem to be doctored; Swanton was unable to identify the plant, but describes it as "a weed a foot high which produces a little yellow fruit just where the leaf comes away from the stalk" and states that it was used for rheumatism and gonorrhea.[100]

27. *Pesē-heleswv*

Swanton translates this as "woman's breast medicine" and states that this is a plant and that the roots were used in a medicine for women with swollen breasts. Swanton gives no plant description or scientific name.[101] It is likely that this term refers to the medicine made for this ailment and not to a plant.

28. *Efolo-heleswv*

Swanton is unable to identify this plant by name. He translates the Mvskoke name as "screech owl medicine" and describes it as a plant found "far out in the woods, growing in small bunches," which was used for eye troubles.[102] Lewis does not use this to identify a plant.

29. *Awvnhē-heleswv*

Swanton was unable to identify this plant, although Caley Proctor described it to him as a plant that grows three feet tall and bears a yellow flower, which is used to cure enlarged spleen.[103]

All the plants and medicines Lewis describes have previously appeared in the written record because Lewis is working from Swanton's published plant list. Thus all these plants have been known to the Mvskoke as medicine plants since at least 1912, the last year Swanton conducted fieldwork for his publication on religion in which they are listed. The uses Swanton attributed to Jackson Lewis would presumably also be known to David Lewis since he learned Jackson Lewis's medicine knowledge. Some of these plants are found much earlier in the written record. *Mēkko-hoyvnēcv* and *passv* are mentioned as early as 1735, in Tchikilli's explanation of the origin of his people to Governor Oglethorpe. *Kvpvpaskv, welanv,* and *vcenv* are mentioned some fifty years later by Hawkins, and *notossv* is mentioned by Bartram. Few medicine plants used in the Southeast prior to removal are found in the written record, even though there was considerable interest in the colony of Georgia in plants that could be marketed for medicinal purposes.[104]

Mvskoke pharmacology changed after removal because of plant availability in the new ecosystem in Indian Territory. The falling away of the taking of the black drink due to the lack of availability of the yaupon plant in Indian Territory is the best documented example of this. The increased documentation of medicine plants in the twentieth century is due to the ethnographers' interest. How many of the plants used after removal to Indian Territory were also used previously is unknown and would of course have depended on their availability in the Southeast. The ability of main *heles-hayv* to see new plant uses through visions would have assured that the Mvskoke would learn how new plants in the new environment were to be used and would have allowed the medicine tradition to continue uninterrupted.

CHAPTER 9: CEREMONIES

Traditional Mvskoke ceremonies are recorded in many written documents. Those most often described were communal ceremonies easily observed by outsiders. One of the earliest ceremonies recorded appeared frequently in the accounts of fur traders, Indian agents, and other non-Mvskoke prior to removal. This was the taking of the black drink by the men of the tribe in the town square. Prior to removal, it appears to have been the custom for men to conduct this ritual daily and/or on occasions when visitors came to the town. The details of these descriptions differ according to the chronicler and to the town. As has already been mentioned, only Hitchcock mentioned this ceremony after removal to Indian Territory.[105]

By far the ceremony most frequently appearing in the written record is the *posketv* (to fast), called in English the Green Corn Ceremony or the Busk. It is held by each ceremonial ground in the summer. This ancient ceremony is at the heart of traditional Mvskoke religion. It was mentioned in the eighteenth-century accounts by Adair, Bossu, Bosomworth, Hall, Bartram, Milfort, Swan, and Hawkins. In the nineteenth century, references to it were included in the writings of Stiggins, Payne, Hitchcock, Tuggle, and Hewitt. In the twentieth century, it is described by ethnographers including Swanton, Speck, Robbins, Howard, Bell, and Innes.[106] Among twentieth-century accounts by Mvskoke, other than those presented through the narrative voices of anthropologists, Susie Foster mentioned the ceremony in the recollections published by her town, Thlopthlocco. In the 1930s several Mvskoke referred to the ceremony in the Indian Pioneer Papers interviews. Samuel Checote provided this description:

During the crop season it was an unwritten law that no one should partake of the roasting ear before a celebration or festival had been held. This ceremony was awe-inspiring as these, ironically speaking, uncivilized Indians were trying to make the Spirit behind these crop miracles happy by showing the Spirit their appreciation.

On the appointed day the Indians would assemble at the . . . ceremonial ground. Beginning early in the morning before break-fast, the men would drink a liquid made up of different kinds of herbs, prepared by the medicine man of the grounds. By drinking the mixture they were cleaning out their system via vomiting. This would be kept up all day with interruptions now and then by games they played.

In the evening just about twilight, the men ran to the nearby stream for a bathing. After spending some time in the water, they return and it is then that they are ready to eat the meal. . . .

After the evening meal, they are ready for the night frolic which lasts all night long, to be completed by the playing of Indian ball. Many phases of this celebration would make a topic of itself. In the night frolics, no one is allowed to go to bed, but there was no rule necessary to that effect as no one wished to do so. Everybody wished to express thanks for the Great Spirit so that he shall always be good to the Indians.[107]

Bose Scott provided another description:

When Indian corn was grown, the ripening of the grain con-stituted an important era in the year. The whole band usually assembled to celebrate this feast.

It was the custom at that time to produce fire by rubbing two sticks together, and the fire thus produced was sent from band to band as a token of friendship.

At the place of assembly a large fire was kept up, and the war-riors and women gathered around it dancing and singing songs of gratitude to the Great Spirit, for sparing them and their friends throughout the year. If famine had overtaken them or many of their people had fallen in battle, then these joyous songs were intermingled with wailing and mournful sounds. . . .

If a criminal escaped from his bonds during the festival and made his way into the charmed circle of the dance, he was considered under the protection of the Great Spirit, and his pardon was secured.[108]

Ada Roach explained:

> In preparation for the Stomp Dances, the strongest young men of the tribe were sent out to gather roots for the medicine used. They weren't to take any tools or comforts with them. They were to sleep on the bare ground and dig the roots with their hands.
>
> The men would go off and drink the medicine on an empty stomach, change clothing after bathing and then sat down to a feast prepared by the women.
>
> At night they began dancing. The men and women each had a leader. The men wore a feather and the women four turtle shells, which contained a few pebbles, on each ankle. The shells aided the tom tom in making music for the dancers. They danced frequently all night.[109]

The Green Corn Ceremony was not the only communal ritual among the Mvskoke. In the twentieth century, accounts by both Mvskoke and non-Mvskoke frequently mention Stomp Dances, referring to other dances similar in form to the Green Corn Ceremony and occurring in the summer season. Some of the authors of these accounts probably include the Green Corn Ceremony as a Stomp Dance. Traditional ball games held in conjunction with the Green Corn Ceremony and the Stomp Dances are ceremonial as well. Accounts of the ball games appeared from the seventeenth through the twentieth centuries. Bell described the entire ceremonial season as it occurred in the early 1980s. The *posketv* occurred in midsummer and a ceremonial ground would hold several other dances from spring to first frost. Squirrel dinners are held during the winter and some ball games between friendly towns might be played on winter Sundays. In the early spring, wild-onion dinners were held to raise money for the summer ceremonies. Since members of ceremonial grounds attended the dances of other grounds, summer weekends were frequently taken up with dances.[110]

The Mvskoke performed other rituals on a contingent basis. The most frequently mentioned of these were those that marked the transition from one stage of life to another, such as birth rituals, naming ceremonies, marriage rituals, and death rituals. Numerous accounts described the naming ceremonies for young males, which took place during the Green Corn Ceremony. A nineteenth-century account of this prior to removal was provided by Stiggins: "At the annual busk young men get their war names to replace the name they have been called since infancy. One of the chiefs or warriors calls out the young man's new name and tells him he can now assume the manners and customs of other men and puts a feather in his head."[111] One hundred years later, an account by Sandy Fife in the Indian Pioneer Papers sounded similar:

> When a young man takes his first medicine as a man at a Green Corn Dance he is given a nickname. . . . Sometimes the name is that of a bird or animal or sometimes a boy is named by his actions while he is taking the medicine. . . . A certain man calls the boy out by the new name. This man is the 'Caller' and the name is long drawn out. He [the boy] goes to that arbor and to those clansmen. Then he is recognized by that name by the king who gives him a gift of tobacco and after that he is always known by that name.[112]

The written record includes few accounts of rituals like those Lewis describes in chapter 8. The Blessing Ceremony and Doctoring a House do not appear in other accounts as they are described by Lewis. There are accounts of attending to a house, like sprinkling a house with medicine after a death.[113] While no accounts of reburial ceremonies are recorded, there are accounts of burials. The burial descriptions differ in details. Prior to removal, it appears that it was common to bury a family member inside the house.[114] Jackson Lewis described this type of burial for his own father in Alabama (chapter 2). After removal, burials occurred in the ground and a small house was erected over the grave.[115] David Lewis's grandmother, Jeanetta Jacobs, was buried in this manner. Traditionally possessions were buried with the deceased.[116]

When contextualized within the written record, it is clear that David Lewis's account both extends and changes the understanding of Mvskoke medicine. He extends the understanding by providing much new detail: parts of a story or sacred narrative that explain the origin of medicines; a description of the selection, training, and initiation of main *heles-hayv*; an explanation of types of medicine people; more knowledge of plant uses; and new descriptions of ceremonies and of the medicine stick. He changes the understanding of the role of medicine schools. Lewis confronts the written record and provides a Mvskoke commentary on its authenticity. He recontextualizes that record by placing it in his own cultural experience. Given the centuries of change that the Mvskoke have experienced and the several different cultural traditions that have come to constitute Mvskoke culture, the many threads of information about Mvskoke religion weave together to present a picture that is multifaceted and contested. New knowledge in some cases brings new understanding and in other cases brings confusion. The confusion, for the most part, cannot be alleviated; the contradictions cannot be reconciled. What remains are many voices speaking from many cultural backgrounds in many time periods. The time is past when earlier accounts can be fully understood and validated. It is clear from Lewis's account that some chroniclers had but a minimal and confused understanding of Mvskoke religion. He suggests that the Mvskoke people have not been forthcoming in committing their sacred traditions to writing and thus what is known to the uninitiated is minimal. He brings into question the value of the many superficial accounts of Mvskoke medicine. Of course, now it is not possible for chroniclers from across the centuries to stand up and explain their points of view, Mvskoke and non-Mvskoke, or the shallowness or depth of their knowledge.

Beyond the clear value of the information he shares and of his insightful contextualization of the previous written record, David Lewis's work is important as the voice of a religious specialist at the beginning of the twenty-first century. He defends the continuation of a centuries-old religious tradition and insists that the tradition be viewed in its sacred, living context rather than as items of information on the printed page. This last emphasis is of value to Mvskoke and non-Mvskoke alike.

APPENDIX C

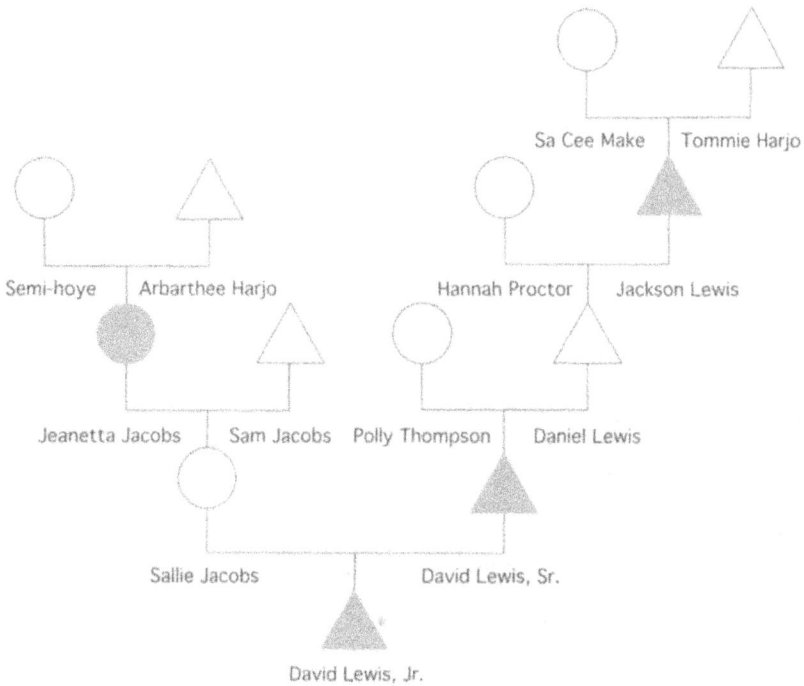

Shading indicates known initiated medicine people

Partial Genealogy of the Lewis and Jacobs Families

GLOSSARY AND PRONUNCIATION GUIDE

While Mvskoke pronunciation is complex, there are four letters which represent sounds quite different than those English speakers expect. English approximations of those sounds are as follows:

c as in English in*ch*
i as in English h*ey*
r as in English fif*th*ly
v as in English *ago*[1]

Akcelvlaskv.	*Betula* sp., white birch.
Akhatkv.	*Platanus occidentalis*, sycamore.
Akwahnv.	Willow.
Awvnhē-heleswv.	Constipation.
Cēpvnvke.	The group of youths.
Coskv.	*Quercus stellata*, post oak.
Cvto-heleswv.	Rock medicine.
Efolo-heleswv.	Screech owl medicine.
Epohfvnkv (Ifofanga).	The One Above.
Haloneske (aloneske).	*Tephrosia virginiana*, devil's shoestring.
Hece-pakpvkē.	*Lobelia* sp., tobacco bloom.
Heles-hayv.	Medicine maker; medicine person.
Heles-hvtke.	*Panax quinquefolium*, ginseng, translates as "white medicine."
Heleswv.	Medicine.
Henehvlke.	Assistants to the chief.
Hesaketvmesē.	Breath holder; master of breath.
Kērrv.	One who knows; a medicine specialist who knows from experience.
Kofockv-rakko.	*Monarda* sp., horsemint.
Kolaswv-holvnwv.	Star shit.
Kvpvpaskv.	*Lindera benzoin*, spicewood or spicebush.
Kvtohwv.	Honey locust.
Mēkko.	King; chief.
Mēkko-hoyvnēcv.	*Salix humilis*, translates as "king passing through"; called "red root" in English.
Mēkkvlke.	The group of chiefs.
Muscogee.	Mvskoke as spelled in English alphabet.
Muskogee.	The language of the Mvskoke; a city in Oklahoma.
Mvskoke.	Traditional spelling of Muscogee.
Mvskokvlke.	The Muscogee people; in this text refers to the Mvskoke people of past times.
Notossv.	*Angelica atropurpurea*.
Owalv.	A medicine specialist who prophesies, like a fortune teller.
Passv.	*Eryngium yuccifolium*, button snake root or bear grass.

Pesē-heleswv.	Woman's breast medicine.
Posketv.	To fast; a name for the Green Corn Ceremony.
Poyvfekcv-heleswv.	Spirit medicine.
Pvkanvho.	*Prunus* sp., wild plum.
Pvrko-rakko.	*Vitis palmata*, big grape or summer grape.
Tartahkv.	*Populus deltoides*, cottonwood.
'To-heleko.	*Phoradendron* sp., mistletoe.
Tvfosho.	*Ulmus* sp., elm.
Tvlwv.	Town.
Tvstvnvke.	The group of warriors.
Vcenv.	Cedar.
Vlv.	*Aesculus* sp., buckeye.
Vsse.	A medicine used prior to removal, called the "black drink" in English.
Vtakrv-lvste.	*Baptisia* sp., black weed.
Welanv.	*Chenopodium ambrosioides*, wormseed.
W⁻eso.	*Sassafras* sp., sassafras.
Yvnvsv-heleswv.	Bison medicine.

NOTES

Preface

1. Crane 1918; Wright 1986:2–4.

Chapter 1

1. Gatschet 1884:244–45. The name of this Mvskoke town is variously spelled Kasihta, Cusseta, and Kvsehtv. Cusseta is used henceforth in this text.

2. Green 1990:17; Wright 1986:xi.

3. Green 1990:17–20; Wright 1986:xi. It is estimated that 90 percent of the aboriginal population of the Southeast may have died as a result of warfare with Europeans and European diseases, like smallpox and measles; see Green 1982: 17 and Smith 1989:63.

4. Swanton (1913, 1915, 1922, 1928a, 1928b, 1931) provides the most extensive accounts of Mvskoke culture, relying on earlier accounts as well as his own fieldwork conducted in the early twentieth century.

5. Green 1982:3–4.

6. Swanton 1928a:191–92.

7. Haas 1945:69.

8. Wright 1986:3–14.

9. Swanton 1928a:114–66; Spoehr 1947:204–7.

10. Swanton provides detail on religion; see 1928b:546–614 for information on the Green Corn Ceremony, 614–21 on *heles-hayv*, 481–98 on supernatural entities, and 538–44 on the ritual of the black drink. An excellent overview of the black drink is found in Fairbanks 1979.

11. Martin 1991:57; Green 1982:28–29; Wood 1989:38. For more on this period see Braund 1993 and Corkran 1967.

12. Wright 1986:133.

13. Woodward (1859:60–65) disputes the assertion that McGillivray's mother was half French. The assertion that she was half French was published by Pickett, who found it in Milfort's (1959) text. Woodward knew McGillivray's last wife and some of his children and understood that McGillivray's mother was full-blood. McGillivray did not have a white person's education. His letters were written for him by a Scot named Alex Leslie.

14. Wright 1986:137–39; Martin 1991:83–84.

15. Milfort 1959. Swanton (1928:324–27) provides an explanation of how McGillivray managed to come to some degree of power in a cultural system that ordinarily would have rejected such an interloper. Woodward (1959:45), reminiscing in 1858 about his lifetime among the Mvskoke, explained that in his experience in the nineteenth century, it was generally the "half-breeds and mixed-bloods" who spoke English and would get "dubbed a chief" by the whites. "The Indians, learning who the whites thought was their leader and not being as ambitious of distinction as the whites generally are, when any talking or compromising is to be done, those persons are put forward." Thus the Indians speaking for the whole were not usually the true leaders.

Most analyses of Creek political history emphasize the importance of towns but neglect the importance of clans. Since strong clan recognition was still found among the Oklahoma Creeks in the 1930s, it is likely that an understanding of clan issues would increase the understanding of internal political issues from contact until at least the beginning of the twentieth century. Spoehr 1947 describes the state of clan allegiance and functions in the 1930s.

16. Cotterill 1954:124–25; Nunez 1958:3–4; Baird 1988:4; Green 1990:53.

17. Woodward (1859:43) provides the Mvskoke name for Jackson.

18. Hawkins 1916: 2,687; Martin 1991:184.

19. Martin 1991:162; Green 1990:55; Woodward 1859:43; Nunez 1958:3–4; Cotterill 1954:124–25. See also Halbert and Ball 1995, a detailed account of the Red Stick War first published in 1895.

20. Green (1982) provides a detailed account of this period.

21. Green 1982:122–25.

22. Green 1982:169–86.

23. Indian Pioneer Papers (hereafter cited as IPP) 5:104–7.

24. IPP 14:410.

25. IPP 52:26.

26. IPP 27:412–13.

27. Green 1982:141–73; Green 1990:83; Hitchcock 1996:121, 157.

28. General Cass, Secretary of War, in a message to the Creeks in January 1832. See Opler 1987.

29. Hitchcock (1996) documented substantial fraudulent behavior in the years after removal. Debo (1989:140) and Opler (1987) discuss this time period.

30. Loughridge and Hodge 1964.

31. IPP 69:444.

32. See May 1996 and Littlefield 1979 for overviews of the history of relations between Africans, African-Americans, and Mvskoke from the colonial period through the 1920s.

33. IPP 44:30.

34. See White and White 1996 for a narrative describing the plight of Opothle Yoholo's group.

35. IPP 52:32–34.

36. White and White 1996; Green 1990:94.

37. Moore 1996:150.

38. See Miner 1989 for a description of these battles in Indian Territory.

39. IPP 65:121.

40. Opler 1987:45.

41. Debo 1989:324–77; Carter 1990:43.

42. IPP 104:60.

43. Opler 1987:48.

44. IPP 51:173.

45. IPP 69:454.

46. Grayson 1988:163–64.

47. Debo 1991:92.

48. Debo 1991:197–98. See also Carter 1999.

49. A lengthy discussion of this case is found in Debo 1991:286, 338–49; Blend 1978.

50. Green 1990:113.

51. Morgan and Morgan 1977:152–54. For more on the politics of the time for the Mvskoke, see Debo 1991. For information about the continued importance of the traditional Mvskoke Creek towns and the Mvskoke response to the new laws, see Opler 1987. For stories recorded from members of the Mvskoke Creek tribe about life in the 1930s, see the Indian Pioneer Papers.

52. Moore 1996:151.

53. Moore 1996:151; http://www.ocevnet.org/creek/myfile.html; Robbins 1976:74–75.

Chapter 2

1. As described in chapter 1, Hitchitee is one of the languages in the Muskogean linguistic family. The members of several southeastern *tvlwv* were Hitchitee speakers, and *tvlwv* were sometimes identified by that name.

2. This refers to the land allotment rolls taken after passage of the Curtis Act. Details like ages and spellings of names are frequently inaccurate on these rolls.

3. The family is mentioned in written documents listed here in chronological order within type.

Accounts by Family Members:

1) David Lewis, Sr.'s handwritten family history, in the personal papers of his son, David Lewis, Jr.

2) David Lewis, Sr., 1937. Indian Pioneer Papers 106:336–40; and 1938, 61:218–21. Lewis was interviewed twice during the Works Progress Administration program to capture oral narrative from Mvskoke.

3) Jerlena King, 1963. Jackson Lewis of the Confederate Creek Regiment. Chronicles of Oklahoma XLI:66–69. Jerlena King is a great granddaughter of Jackson Lewis and is a local historian and writer from Eufaula, Oklahoma.

4) Robert Johnson Perry and Chester Scott, 1998. *Life with the Little People*. Greenfield Center, N.Y.: Greenfield Review Press. Chester Scott, a great grandson of Jackson Lewis, is a member of the Raccoon Clan and was raised in Eufaula, Oklahoma. He is a writer and an artist.

5) Interview with David Lewis, Sr., in the Muskogee Daily Phoenix.

6) Interview with David Lewis, Jr., in Oklahoma Today.

7) Letters about David Lewis, Jr., in the Muscogee Nation News.

Archival Sources and Government Documents:

1) The earliest of these is a Creek census taken in 1832 by Parson and Abbott. This list is organized by tribal town and within each town by name of male head of family. It lists the number of males, females, and slaves for each family.

2) The Dunn Roll of 1867 for Canadian Ufaula lists citizens of the Creek Nation to whom payments were made as a result of the Treaty of June 14, 1866. Each citizen received $17.34.

3) U.S. Senate, Executive Document 198, 1st sess., 59th Cong., 1888. This document contains the "Stidham Roll" of 1886. This roll, prepared by G. W. Stidham, special agent, lists the names of Creek Indians who emigrated at their own expense from the old Creek Nation in Alabama

to the Creek Nation, Indian Territory. These individuals were entitled to repayment for their expenses by the 1832 treaty. While the roll is usually associated with the date 1886, that is the year Agent Owen returned it with proofs of authenticity to the Department of the Interior. Owen had a copy of the roll in 1885; thus Stidham collected it in 1885 or earlier.

4) The 1890 census roll for Muscogee Nation.

5) The 1895 census roll for Eufaula Canadian Town, and for Hickory Ground in Muscogee Nation.

6) The Dawes Enrollment Cards dating from around 1902. These were filled out for all members of the Creeks living at that time and list their tribal towns, both parents by name, and the parents' tribal towns.

7) Testimony regarding allotment made in 1901 and 1902 by Jackson Lewis and Nancy Lewis found in Dawes Enrollment Cards, accompanying materials.

8) Sworn testimony in the "Arbuckle and Gambler" case, taken in 1915, found in Dawes Enrollment Cards, accompanying materials. This is the document that explains the double allotments of the two children, Millie and Tommie Gambler, who were erroneously counted as the children of Arbuckle.

9) A legal document entitled "Proof of Death and Heirship" concerning Jackson Lewis's death in 1910, dated 1960.

Anthropologists' Research:

1) These works include references to Jackson Lewis.
   Swanton, John R.
      Unpublished Field Notes, Anthropological Archives, Smithsonian. Washington, D.C.
      1922. Early History of the Creeks and their Neighbors. Bureau of American Ethnology Bulletin no. 73.
      1928a. Social Organization and Social Usages of the Indians of the Creek Confederacy. Bureau of American Ethnology. Annual Report 42:23–472.
      1928b. Religious Beliefs and Medical Practices of the Creek Indians. Bureau of American Ethnology. Annual Report 42: 474–672.

2) These works include references to Jeanetta Jacobs.
   Spoehr, Alexander
      Unpublished Field Notes, Newberry Library, Chicago, Illinois.
      1947. Changing Kinship Systems: A Study in the Acculturation of the Creeks, Cherokee, and Choctaw. Chicago: Field Museum of Natural History, Anthropological Series 33: 151–235.

Other Records:
   Some Pumpkins on Speaking Creek. *Muskogee Times-Democrat*, Sept. 9, 1908.

4. Dawes enrollment card of Jackson Lewis.
5. King 1963:66; Swanton 1928a:395.
6. Swanton 1928a:395.

7. Perry and Scott 1998:3–9. King (1963:66), in her article on Jackson Lewis, mentions the death of his father in Alabama, Jackson wearing out his shoes walking, and that he almost lost his life crossing the Mississippi when the pony he was riding was swept from under him.

There is confusion about Jackson's age when the migration occurred. King lists his age as either six or nine; Scott lists it as seven. The Stidham Roll lists him as six years of age. As David Lewis mentions, exact ages are very difficult to determine for Mvskoke individuals in the nineteenth century. What is known is that Jackson was old enough to remember walking, riding the pony, and nearly being swept away, but was apparently still a small child.

While Perry and Scott (1998) spell Jackson Lewis's name Jock-O-Gee, David Lewis, Sr., in his handwritten family history, spells it Cakoccee, and King (1963:68) spells it Cakoce. That Jackson Lewis had the name Jack as a small boy comes from the account of this story by Perry and Scott. King also translates the name as "little Jack" but does not explain how it was received. Lewis, Sr., does not translate the name.

8. U.S. Senate, Executive Document 198, 1st sess., 50th Cong. The "(m)" stands for male.

9. David Lewis, Sr., IPP 61:226–27.

10. Ibid.

11. David Lewis, Sr., IPP 106:339.

12. This information appears on Jackson Lewis's tombstone.

13. Perry and Scott 1998:11.

14. King 1963:68. This was an important battle for the Mvskoke during the Civil War.

15. David Lewis, Sr., IPP 106:340.

16. David Lewis, Sr., IPP 61:228–29; 106:339–40.

17. Swanton 1928a:102.

18. Loughridge and Hodge (1964) provide the alphabet. The spelling Lahta Yahola is found in King 1963:66. King explains that it was probably a Creek war name and states that as he grew to manhood, Jackson Lewis received three titles or names entitling him to a change of seat in the Eufaula Square Ground.

19. National Archives, Southwest Division, Fort Worth, Tex., Dunn Roll, 1867; Creek Census, 1890; Creek Census, 1895; Allotment Roll Cards, Creek Indians. U.S. Senate, Executive Document 198, 1st sess., 50th Cong.

20. David Lewis, Sr., handwritten account; King 1963:68. Perry and Scott (1999:12) state that Jackson Lewis married Nancy Phillips.

21. King 1963:66–69; Creek Papers, Oklahoma Historical Society.

22. *Muskogee Times-Democrat*, Sept. 9, 1908.

23. Swanton 1928a:32, 147, 436.

24. Swanton 1928b.

25. King 1963:69.

26. *Muskogee Daily Phoenix*.

27. David Lewis, Sr., handwritten account; Muskogee Daily Phoenix.

28. *Muskogee Daily Phoenix*.

29. National Archives, Southwest Division, Fort Worth, Tex., Creek Census, 1890; Allotment Roll Cards, Creek Indians; Sworn Testimony in the Arbuckle and Gambler case taken in 1915.

30. Linda Collins, IPP 65:272; Mary Freeman, IPP 63:80.
31. Spoehr, Unpublished Field Notes, Newberry Library, Chicago, Illinois; Spoehr 1947:151–235.
32. McDermott 1993:70.
33. Bar 1992:12.
34. Platt 1993:2.
35. McDermott 1993:62.

Chapter 4

1. As described in this chapter the selection process involves a test performed at the birth of the candidate by the medicine person looking for a replacement. Candidates are usually kin of the medicine person. Newborn infants are tested to see if they have the right character to become a medicine person. In Lewis's case, there were two medicine persons in his matrilocal household searching for the right infant, and both decided to test him at birth. Each prepared medicine when it was time for the birth. If the baby did not arrive in four days, the medicine had to be thrown away and a new portion made. To throw the old medicine away, the chants are removed from it and the water and plants then thrown away.

Further, selection is a comprehensive learning experience, and was the focus of Lewis's childhood. He uses a description of his own training as an example of the manner in which main *heles-hayv* trained their replacements. For the infant who passes the test and is chosen, the training process begins immediately. While a newborn is obviously not ready to receive instruction, the infant immediately begins receiving medicine. The actual training begins almost immediately with the teaching of the medicine plants and of "the story," the esoteric knowledge which explains the origin of medicine (parts of it make up chapter 6). After this information is mastered, the child is initiated. In Lewis's case, this occurred at approximately six years of age. After initiation, the child is taught the words to the chants and instructed in the manner in which he or she is to acquire tunes for the chants. Once the young *heles-hayv* has learned the words and acquired the tunes, he is given his first medicine stick and is ready to make medicine. The training process is thus complete by the time the initiate is nine or ten years of age.

The story of the Holy Man selecting a young boy to train as his sole replacement is told in chapter 6. It sets the pattern for each initiated medicine person to follow in the selection and training of his or her single replacement. The trainee never asks to be trained. Instead, the medicine person selects someone to train. In this story, the Holy Man "knew" that the boy was the type who would not misuse his power. This was important since the boy must learn destructive as well as constructive powers. He would be able to harm as well as help people, but the intention is that the medicine person does not put these negative powers to use.

Medicine people looked for a sign that a newborn baby was special. For example, a baby born with his or her face still covered with membrane was thought to have the potential to be a great medicine person or a fortune-teller. The Holy Man could tell by looking if a person was to be chosen, but the medicine people would have to test people to know if they would ever misuse what was going to be given to them. Once you have made up your mind to test a baby, once you have chosen the mother, you make the medicine and wait for the baby to be born. If the baby is not born in four days, if the medicine is not used by the fourth day, you will make a new batch. Once you have made the medicine, it cannot be thrown out. The chants are removed or taken back and the roots and water are then thrown away. Any medicine made by a medicine person is to be used within four days and used for four days. When the baby is born, the medicine is given to the baby to drink to see what kind of a person that baby will be in fifty or sixty years. The baby being tested will take that medicine as if a big thirst has come over him or her. Then you will know that this is a chosen person to carry on as your replacement. A medicine person does not come into full power until the age of fifty or sixty and the test tells what kind of person he or she will be then.

2. When Lewis was approximately six years of age, his father and grandmother determined that he was ready to be initiated. Since each had selected him to carry on their unique power and knowledge, each initiated him separately. The initiations Lewis describes are similar although the times of year differed. He was initiated in the winter by his father and in the summer by his grandmother. He explains that a medicine person must initiate his or her candidate in the season that is the opposite of the season of his own initiation. Thus Lewis's father, initiated in the summer, had to initiate him in the winter. His grandmother was initiated in winter and thus had to initiate him in the summer. Having thus been initiated in both summer and winter, Lewis has the choice of initiating his own successor in either season. He also has the option of training two infants.

3. The young initiate now has the full powers of a main *heles-hayv*. His training is not yet finished, however. It is not until after initiation that he is taught the words to the medicine chants. A *heles-hayv* teaches his novice the words but not the tunes to the medicine chants. The tunes are not passed down. Instead, each new young *heles-hayv* must find his own tunes.

4. Lewis's grandmother and father were trained by different medicine people who were from different *tvlwv* and probably spoke different Muskogean languages. It is understandable that the chants would be different.

5. At this point, the young initiate is ready to make his first medicine. He has learned the story of how the medicine began, learned the plants and their uses, and the words to the chants. He has been initiated and found his own tunes for the chants. In order to make medicine, however, he must have a medicine stick. The stick is the tool of Mvskoke medicine people. It is used to push the sacred words into the medicine.

6. Lewis's father and grandmother assured him they would always be there to give him advice and help. While both are now deceased, they continue to communicate with him in his dreams.

Chapter 6

1. This is the medicine person's marriage ceremony. It takes place in the sacred ground. A medicine person cannot divorce.

2. The words are washed as you sing them when you sweat. When you sit in your sacred ground, the words are not washed and purified; they are only washed and purified when you sing them in the sweat house. Water carries away impurities of the body. If you give a person medicine to make them throw up and cleanse the impurities out of their bodies, we have them throw up in running water. If the people see anything unusual—a feather lying on the porch, anything unusual that normally does not belong—they wrap it up and take it to running water, and

running water will kill anything that is evil that has been put on the feather.

3. So this part of the story shows how the medicine people are in partnership with nature. We always treat plants with respect and use sacred words before we remove them from the ground. When the main *heles-hayv* is shown a new cure, there is an order to the visions. First, we see the plant, see it grow from a seedling to full grown and then death. Next we are shown the symptoms of the sickness the plant is used to cure. Last we get the words to the chant. This is why I say, the main *heles-hayv* does not learn new cures by trial and error. He or she is shown the cures through visions.

Chapter 8

1. The first day you use most, but not all, of the medicine in jar number one. Then you pour the medicine in jar number two out into jar one until the level of the medicine in jar two is down to the mark on jar two indicating day two. The second day, you again use most, but not all of the medicine in jar one and then refill it from jar two, emptying jar two down to the mark for day three. After using most of the medicine in jar one on day three, you refill jar one with the remaining medicine in jar two. The fourth day you use all the medicine in jar one.

Chapter 9

1. The four sacred poles mark the corners of a square about ten feet long and five feet wide. This square serves as my sacred ground for this ceremony. I set it up on the grounds outside the council house.

Appendix A

1. See Gatschet 1884:235–51 and Swanton 1928a:33–68 for a discussion of the Tchikilli legend.

2. Nairne 1988; Adair 1930; Bosomworth 1958; Bossu 1962; Hall Manuscript, Creek Papers, Gilcrease Institute Archives.

3. Adair 1930:490. See also Wright 1986:132 and Williams 1930:vii–xxx.

4. Wright 1986:30, 132; Martin 1991:17; Waselkov and Braund 1995:1–23.

5. Bartram 1995: Giver and Taker Away of the Breath of Life 119, 143; belief in shamanic powers to change the weather and cure sickness 145; religious specialists the "High Priest and Juniors in every Town or Tribe" 118, 123, 147; belief in an afterlife and in the Soul 149; description of the busk or "first fruits feast" 125, 507–8; descriptions, with botanical names of plants used as medicines 161–64.

6. Waselkov and Braund 1995:16.

7. A misuse of the term *tvstvnvke*.

8. Milfort 1959: drinking of the black drink 123–24, 139; Green Corn "harvest" festival 134–35.

9. Milfort 1959:138.

10. Swan 1855:257, 258.

11. Swan 1855: funeral rituals 265, 270; the black drink ceremony 266–67; diseases, medicine cures, and medicine people 270–71; and ceremonial dances 277.

12. Hawkins 1848: description of the Green Corn Ceremony 75–78; Ceremony initiating Youth into Manhood 78–79; medicine making 77; medicines 79–80; afterlife 80; Hawkins 1916: black drink 32, 222, 431.

13. Hawkins 1848:75, 78.

14. Ibid.:75–79.

15. Stiggins 1989:51–64.

16. Ibid.:60.

17. Ibid.:49, 53.

18. Spoehr 1947:165; Wyman 1989:13–20, 143; Woodward 1859:6–7.

19. Swanton 1932:172; Payne 1932:172–95; quotes from Payne 1932:194, 195, 185.

20. Hitchcock 1996: origin story 123–26; medicine practices 137; witchcraft 139; and burial customs 129.

21. Hitchcock 1996:115; Fairbanks 1979:139. Hitchcock later served as secretary of the interior during the allotment process in Indian Territory. Of his leadership, Debo (1991:61) wrote: "Hitchcock made an honest attempt to guard the tribal property from the predatory private interests that began to snatch it as soon as the tribal control was released; but he never grasped the elemental fact that he was administering four great estates belonging to a hundred thousand individuals, rather than the public domain."

22. Woodhouse 1992:103, 156, 159.

23. Grayson 1988: naming ceremony for male youth 22–23; Indian war medicine which some of the men in his regiment used during the Civil War to protect themselves against injury 102.

24. Tuggle 1973:55, 56, 64, 73; quotes 73, 74.

25. Sturtevant (1987) provides a review of anthropological materials on the Mvskoke.

26. Gatschet 1884:vi; Hinsley (1981:176–80) provides an account of Gatschet's life and relationship with the Bureau of American Ethnology.

27. Gatschet 1884: "holder of breath" and other "genii and mythic animals" 215–16; an initiation into manhood 158–59; and a description of the Green Corn Ceremony 177–83.

28. Hewitt 1939:119–59.

29. Littlefield 1993:6–7; Riley 1985:46–49; Posey 1993.

30. Speck 1907, 1911.

31. Swanton 1928b.

32. Perdue 1993; IPP.

33. Opler 1987:31.

34. Spoehr 1941, 1947; Spoehr Field Notes, Field Museum.

35. Sturtevant 1988:110. While the Florida Seminoles were also part of the Creek Confederacy prior to removal and their flight south into present-day Florida, the major twentieth-century works on their religion, like Greenlee and Sturtevant, are not included here. There are many similarities in religion among the Florida Seminoles and the Oklahoma Seminoles and Creeks, but there are also differences, and thus the twentieth-century religious descriptions have been limited to Oklahoma.

36. Robbins 1976; Howard and Lena 1984; Sattler 1987; Bell 1984, 1990.

37. Thlopthlocco Tribal Town 1978.

38. Oliver 1985.

39. Bear Heart with Larkin 1998.

40. Perry and Scott 1998:ix, x.

Appendix B

1. Bossu 1962:149.
2. Hall manuscript:6.
3. Swan 1855:270–71.
4. Waselkov and Braund 1995:118.
5. Hewitt 1939:146.
6. Ibid.:156.
7. Speck 1907:121.
8. Swanton 1928a:367, 1928b:614–17, 638, 711.
9. IPP 13:440.
10. IPP 24:245–46.
11. Thlopthlocco Tribal Town 1978:1.
12. Bell 1984:106; 1990:336.
13. Swanton [1946]1979:714.
14. Timberlake 1927; Mooney 1900.
15. IPP 49:390.
16. Swanton 1928b:620.
17. Speck 1911:211–12.
18. Hewitt 1939; Swanton 1928b.
19. Hewitt 1939:155.
20. Swanton 1928b:620.
21. Hawkins 1848.
22. Swanton 1928b:620–21.
23. Ibid.:617–18.
24. Howard and Lena 1984:21.
25. Bear Heart with Larkin 1998.
26. Adair 1775:122, quoted in Swanton 1928b:627–28.
27. Swanton 1928a:248.
28. Swanton 1928b:617.
29. Speck 1907:122–33, 1911:215–35.
30. Howard and Lena 1984:74, 76, 80.
31. Speck 1911:212.
32. Swanton 1928b:628.
33. Howard and Lena 1984:23.
34. Posey 1993; Littlefield 1993; Wofford 1999.
35. *Indian Journal*, Oct. 31, 1902.
36. IPP 32:182–84.
37. Hewitt 1939:154.
38. Swanton 1928a:511.
39. Grayson 1988; Thlopthlocco Tribal Town 1978; Perry and Scott 1998; Lomawaima 1987; Oliver 1985; Bear Heart with Larkin 1998; IPP.
40. IPP 66:460–61.
41. Swanton 1928b:496–97.
42. Ibid.:649.
43. Howard and Lena 1984:211.
44. Oliver 1985:4; Perry and Scott 1998.
45. IPP 33:42.
46. IPP 52:365.

47. Gatschet 1884:235–51.
48. Swanton 1928a:33–68.
49. Gatschet 1884:246.
50. Hawkins 1848:81–83; Gatschet 1884:222.
51. Waselkov and Braund 1995:42.
52. Hitchcock 1996:123–26.
53. Swanton 1928b:546–47.
54. Swanton 1928a:65.
55. Speck 1911:211.
56. Swanton 1928b.
57. Howard and Lena 1984.
58. Swanton 1928b:655.
59. Bell 1984:211.
60. IPP 13:415.
61. Swanton 1928b:639, 640, 642, 650–52, 655.
62. Speck 1911:220.
63. Swanton 1928b:642.
64. IPP 13:441.
65. Swanton 1928b:655; Fairbanks 1979:140.
66. Howard and Lena 1984:42–45.
67. IPP 15:27.
68. Swanton 1928b:639, 640, 655.
69. Howard and Lena 1984:29–32, 136–38.
70. Swan 1853:268; Hawkins 1848:78–79.
71. Swanton 1928b:655–56.
72. Ibid.:653, 656, 648; Howard and Lena 1984:64; IPP 34:166.
73. Swanton 1928b:657; Bartram 1995:47; Howard and Lena 1984:62.
74. Hawkins 1848:77; Howard and Lena 1984:52–53; Swanton 1928b:657.
75. Swanton 1928b:639, 644, 649, 657.
76. IPP 9:123.
77. Hawkins 1848:77.
78. Howard and Lena 1984:61.
79. Swanton 1928b:649, 650, 652, 657.
80. Ibid.:650, 657; Howard and Lena 1984:39–40; IPP 13:441.
81. Swanton 1928b:658.
82. Ibid.:658, 647.
83. IPP 15:59.
84. Ibid.:53, 52:340, 65:268, for examples.
85. Swanton 1928b:568, 647, 662.
86. Ibid.:658; IPP 14:471.
87. Swanton 1928b:658.
88. Ibid.
89. Ibid.:659, 649.
90. Ibid.:645, 649, 659.
91. Ibid.:659.
92. Ibid.:645, 649, 659.
93. Ibid.:649, 650, 659.
94. Ibid.:649, 650.

95. Ibid.:660; IPP 34:166.
96. Swanton 1928b:645, 649, 660; Howard and Lena 1984:26.
97. Swanton 1928b:660.
98. Ibid.:641, 647, 650; Howard and Lena 1984:55.
99. Swanton 1928b:650, 653, 662; Howard and Lena 1984:59.
100. Swanton 1928b:661.
101. Ibid.:662.
102. Ibid.
103. Ibid.
104. Vogle 1990:71–75.
105. Fairbanks (1979) provided a detailed discussion of this drink.
106. Adair 1930 Argument VII; Bossu 1962:147; Bosomworth 1958:272, 280, 288–90; Hall manuscript:8; Bartram 1995b 125, 507–8; Milfort 1959:134–35; Swan 1855:267–68; and Hawkins 1848:75–78. In the nineteenth century, accounts were included in the writings of Stiggins 1989:51–64; Payne 1932:172–95; Hitchcock 1996:132–37; Tuggle 1973:64; and Hewitt 1939:150–54. In the twentieth century, it is described by ethnographers including Swanton 1928b; Speck 1907:137–45; Robbins 1976:143–48; Howard and Lena 1984:123–56; Bell 1984:157–97; and Innes 1997:163–75.
107. IPP 2:23–24.
108. IPP 43:477–78.
109. IPP 52:344.
110. Bell 1984:158–59.
111. Stiggins 1989:64.
112. IPP 14:256.
113. Speck 1907:119.
114. Hall manuscript:9.
115. Hitchcock 1996:129; Speck 1907:119.
116. Hitchcock 1996:129; IPP 65:121.

Glossary and Pronunciation Guide
1. See Martin and Mauldin 2000:xvii–xxii for a more thorough explanation of pronunciation.

Bibliography

Archival Sources

Oklahoma Historical Society, Oklahoma City, Okla.
Creek National Records.
Works Progress Administration, Indian Pioneer History Project for
Oklahoma. Grant Foreman, Director. Identified in text as Indian
Pioneer Papers (IPP). Includes interviews with David Lewis, Sr.,
1937–38, vol. 61:218–21; vol. 106:336–40. Oklahoma Historical
Society. Oklahoma City, Okla.

Thomas Gilcrease Institute of American History and Art Library. Tulsa, Okla.
Creek Papers, 1783–1892.
Hall Manuscript. 1775 Creek Papers.

National Archives, Southwest Division. Fort Worth, Tex.
1832 Creek Census by Parson and Abbott.
1867 Dunn Roll, Creek Nation.
1890 Census Roll for Creek Nation.
1895 Census Roll for Creek Nation.
1902 Dawes Commission Enrollment Cards for Creek Nation and
accompanying materials.

Hawkins, Benjamin
1798–1799 Sketch of Creek Country. Handwritten copy given to Thomas
Jefferson. American Philosophical Society. Philadelphia, Pa.

Hewitt, J. N. B.
1881–1882 Muskhogean Sociological Material obtained from L. C.
Perryman. Smithsonian Institution National Anthropological Archives.
Washington, D.C.

Swanton, John
Creek Ethnographic and Vocabulary Notes. Smithsonian Institution
National Anthropological Archives. Washington, D.C.

Spoehr, Alexander
Field Notes. Field Museum of Natural History. Department of
Anthropology Archives. Chicago, Ill.

Newspapers

Indian Journal. Eufaula, Okla.
Muscogee Nation News. Okmulgee, Okla.
Muskogee Daily Phoenix. Muskogee, Okla.
Muskogee Times-Democrat. Muskogee, Okla.

Private Papers of David Lewis, Jr.

Office of Superintendent of the Five Civilized Tribes
1960   Proof of Death and Heirship of Jackson Lewis.
Lewis, David, Sr.
n.d.   Handwritten Family History.

Theses and Dissertations

Bell, Amelia Rector
1984   "Creek Ritual: the Path to Peace." Ph.D. diss., University of Chicago.
Blend, Benay
1978   "Jackson Barnett and the Oklahoma Indian Probate System." Master's thesis, University of Texas at Arlington.
Innes, Pamela Joan
1997   "From One to Many, From Many to One: Speech Communities in the Muskogee Stompdance Population." Ph.D. diss., University of Oklahoma.
Robbins, Lester
1976   "The Persistence of Traditional Religious Practices among the Creek Indians." Ph.D. diss., Southern Methodist University.
Sattler, Richard Allen
1987   "*Seminoli Italwa*: Socio-Political Change among the Oklahoma Seminoles between Removal and Allotment, 1836–1905." Ph.D. diss., University of Oklahoma.

Electronic Sources

Creek Nation
1999   Web Page http://www.ocevnet.org/creek/myfile.html.

Government Documents

Executive Document 198, U.S. Senate, 1st sess., 59th Cong.
1888   Stidham Roll of 1868, Creek Nation.

Books, Pamphlets, Articles

Adair, James
1930   *The History of the American Indians.* Edited by Samuel Cole Williams. Johnson City, Tenn.: The Watauga Press.
Baird, W. David, ed.
1988   *A Creek Warrior for the Confederacy: The Autobiography of Chief G. W. Grayson.* Norman: University of Oklahoma Press.
Bar, Deanne
1992   Letter to the editor. *Muscogee Nation News* 12.

Bartram, William
1995a   Observations on the Creek and Cherokee Indians. In *William Bartram*
         on the Southeastern Indians, edited by G. A. Waselkov and K. E. Braund.
         Lincoln: University of Nebraska Press.
1995b   Travels through North and South Carolina, Georgia, East and West
         Florida. In *William Bartram on the Southeastern Indians*, edited by G.
         A. Waselkov and K. E. Braund. Lincoln: University of Nebraska Press.
Bear Heart, and Molly Larkin
1998   *The Wind Is My Mother*. New York: Berkley Books.
Bell, Amelia Rector
1990   Separate People: Speaking of Creek Men and Women. *American*
         Anthropologist 92:332–45.
Bosomworth, Thomas
1958   Journal of Thomas Bosomworth. In *Documents relating to Indian*
         Affairs, May 21, 1750–August 7, 1754, edited by William L. McDowell,
         Jr. Columbia, S.C.: South Carolina Archives Department.
Bossu, Jean Bernard
1962   *Jean-Bernard Bossu's Travels in the Interior of North America,*
         1751–1762. Edited by Seymour Feiler. Norman: University of
         Oklahoma Press.
Braund, Kathryn E. Holland
1993   *Deerskins and Duffels: The Creek Indian Trade with Anglo-America,*
         1685–1815. Lincoln: University of Nebraska Press.
Champagne, Duane
1992   *Social Order and Political Change: Constitutional Governments among*
         the Cherokee, the Choctaw, the Chickasaw, and the Creek. Stanford,
         Calif.: Stanford University Press.
Corkran, David H.
1967   *The Creek Frontier, 1540–1783*. Norman: University of Oklahoma Press.
Cotterill, R. S.
1954   *The Southern Indians: The Story of the Civilized Tribes before Removal*.
         Norman: University of Oklahoma Press.
Crane, Verner W.
1918   The Origin of the Name of the Creek Indians. *Journal of American*
         History 5:339–42.
Debo, Angie
1989   *The Road to Disappearance: A History of the Creek Indians*. Norman:
         University of Oklahoma Press.
1991   *And Still the Waters Run: The Betrayal of the Five Civilized Tribes*.
         Princeton, N.J.: Princeton University Press.
Fairbanks, Charles H.
1979   The Function of Black Drink among the Creeks. In *Black Drink:*
         A Native American Tea, edited by C. M. Hudson. Athens: University
         of Georgia Press.
Gatschet, Albert S.
1884   *A Migration Legend of the Creek Indians, with a Linguistic, Historic*
         and Ethnographic Introduction. Philadelphia: D. G. Brinton.

Grayson, Chief G. W.
1988   *A Creek Warrior for the Confederacy*. Edited by David W. Baird. Norman: University of Oklahoma Press.

Green, Michael D.
1982   *The Politics of Indian Removal: Creek Government and Society in Crisis*. Lincoln: University of Nebraska Press.
1990   *The Creeks*. New York: Chelsea House.

Greenlee, Robert
1944   Medicine and Curing Practices of the Modern Florida Seminole. *American Anthropologist* 46:317–28.

Haas, Mary R.
1945   Dialects of the Muskogee Language. *International Journal of American Linguistics* 11:69–74 (repr. in Sturtevant 1987).

Halbert, H. S., and T. H. Ball
1995   *The Creek War of 1813 and 1814*. Tuscaloosa, Ala.: University of Alabama Press (originally published 1895).

Hawkins, Benjamin
1848   A Sketch of the Creek Country, in the Years 1798 and 1799. In *A Combination of A Sketch of the Creek Country, in the Years 1798 and 1799 and Letters of Benjamin Hawkins 1796–1806*. Spartanburg, S.C.: The Reprint Company, 1982.
1916   Letters of Benjamin Hawkins, 1796–1806. In *A Combination of A Sketch of the Creek Country, in the Years 1798 and 1799 and Letters of Benjamin Hawkins 1796–1806*. Spartanburg, S.C.: The Reprint Company, 1982.

Hewitt, J. N. B.
1939   Notes on the Creek Indians. *Bureau of American Ethnology Bulletin Series* 123:119–59.

Hinsley, Curtis M.
1981   *The Smithsonian and the American Indian: Making a Moral Anthropology in Victorian America*. Washington, D.C.: Smithsonian Institution Press.

Hitchcock, Ethan Allen
1996   *A Traveler in Indian Territory: The Journal of Ethan Allen Hitchcock*. Edited by Grant Foreman. Norman: University of Oklahoma Press.

Howard, James, and Willie Lena
1984   *Oklahoma Seminoles: Medicines, Magic, and Religion*. Norman: University of Oklahoma Press.

King, Jerlena
1963   Jackson Lewis of the Confederate Creek Regiment. *The Chronicles of Oklahoma* 41:66–69.

Littlefield, Daniel F., Jr.
1979   *Africans and Creeks: From the Colonial Period to the Civil War*. Westport, Conn.: Greenwood Press.
1992   *Alex Posey: Creek Poet, Journalist, and Humorist*. Lincoln: University of Nebraska Press.
1993   Introduction. In *The Fus Fixico Letters*, by A. Posey. Lincoln: University of Nebraska Press.

Lomawaima, K. Tsianina
1987   Oral Histories from Chilocco Indian Agricultural School: 1920–1940. *American Indian Quarterly* 11:214–54.
Loughridge, R. M., and David M. Hodge
1964   *English and Muskokee Dictionary.* Okmulgee, Okla.: Baptist Home Mission Board.
Martin, Jack B., and Margaret McKane Mauldin
2000   *A Dictionary of Creek/Muskogee, with Notes on the Florida and Oklahoma Seminole Dialects of Creek.* Studies in the Anthropology of North American Indians. Lincoln/London: University of Nebraska Press.
Martin, Joel W.
1991   *Sacred Revolt: The Muskogees' Struggle for a New World.* Boston: Beacon Press.
May, Katja
1996   *African Americans and Native Americans in the Creek and Cherokee Nations, 1830s to 1920s: Collision and Collusion.* New York: Garland Publishing.
McDermott, Maura
1993   Healing from the Earth: How Native Americans Dug Up the Roots of Modern Medicine. *Oklahoma Today.* May–June:62–70.
Milfort, Louis LeClerc
1959   *Memoirs, or a Quick Glance at My Various Travels and My Sojourn in the Creek Nation.* Edited by Ben C. McCary. Kennesaw, Ga.: Continental Book Company.
Miner, Craig H.
1989   *The Corporation and the Indian: Tribal Sovereignty and Industrial Civilization in Indian Territory, 1865–1907.* Norman: University of Oklahoma Press.
Mooney, James
1900   *Myths of the Cherokee.* Volume 19. Washington, D.C.: Annual Report of the Bureau of American Ethnology.
Moore, John
1996   Creek/Mvskoke. In *Native America in the Twentieth Century,* edited by M. B. Davis, 150–52. New York: Garland Publishing.
Morgan, H. Wayne, and Anne Hodges Morgan
1977   *Oklahoma: A Bicentennial History.* New York: W. W. Norton and Company.
Nairne, Thomas
1988   *Nairne's Muskhogean Journals: The 1708 Expedition to the Mississippi River.* Jackson: University Press of Mississippi.
Nunez, Theron A.
1958   Creek Nativism and the Creek War of 1813–1814. *Ethnohistory* 5:1–47,131–75,292–301 (repr. in Sturtevant 1987).
Oliver, Lewis
1985   *Estiyt Omayat = Creek Writings.* Muskogee, Okla.: Bacone College.
Opler, Morris E.
1987   Report on the History and Contemporary State of Aspects of Creek Social Organization and Government, 1937. In *A Creek Sourcebook,* edited by William Sturtevant. New York: Garland Publishing.

Payne, John Howard
1932   The Green Corn Dance. *Chronicles of Oklahoma* 10:170–95.
Perdue, Theda
1993   *Nations Remembered: An Oral History of the Cherokees, Chickasaws,
        Choctaws, Creeks, and Seminoles in Oklahoma, 1865–1907.* Norman:
        University of Oklahoma Press (originally published by Greenwood Press:
        1980).
Perry, Robert Johnson, and Chester Scott
1998   *Life with the Little People.* New York: Greenfield Review Press.
Platt, Mrs. H. Craig
1993   Medicine Man Praised for Healing. *The Muscogee Nation News.* July:2.
Posey, Alexander Lawrence
1993   *The Fus Fixico Letters.* Lincoln: University of Nebraska Press.
Riley, Sam G.
1985   Indian Journal, Voice of Creek Tribe, Now Oklahoma's Oldest
        Newspaper. *Journalism Quarterly* 59(1):46–51, 183.
Smith, Buckingham, ed.
1968   *Narratives of De Soto in the Conquest of Florida.* Gainesville, Fla.:
        Palmetto Press.
Smith, Marvin T.
1989   Aboriginal Population Movements in the Early Historic Period Interior
        Southeast. In *Powhatan's Mantle*, edited by P. H. Wood, G. A. Waselkov,
        and T. M. Hatley. Lincoln: University of Nebraska Press.
Speck, Frank G.
1907   The Creek Indians of Taskigi Town. *Memoirs of the American
        Anthropological Association* 2:99–164.
1911   Ceremonial Songs of the Creek and Yuchi Indians. *University of
        Pennsylvania Museum, Anthropological Publications* 1:157–245.
Spoehr, Alexander
1941   Creek Inter-town Relations. *American Anthropologist* 43:132–33
        (repr. in Sturtevant 1987).
1947   Changing Kinship Systems: A Study in the Acculturation of the Creeks,
        Cherokee, and Choctaw. *Field Museum of Natural History Anthro-
        pological Series,* 33(4):151–235.
Stiggins, George
1989   *Creek Indian History: A Historical Narrative of the Genealogy,
        Traditions and Downfall of the Ispocoga or Creek Indian Tribe of
        Indians, by one of the Tribe.* Edited by Virginia Pounds Brown.
        Birmingham, Ala.: Birmingham Public Library Press.
Sturtevant, William C.
1988   Creek into Seminole. In *Native American Indians in Historical
        Perspective*, edited by E. B. Leacock and N. O. Lurie, 92–128. Prospect
        Heights, Ill.: Waveland Press.
Sturtevant, William C., ed.
1987   *A Creek Source Book.* New York: Garland Publishing.

Swan, Caleb
1855   Topical History: Position and State of Manners and Arts in the Creek,
         or Muscogee Nation in 1791. In *Information respecting the History,
         Condition and Prospects of the Indian Tribes of the United States*, edited
         by H. R. Schoolcraft, 251–83. Vol. 5. Philadelphia: J. B. Lippincott and
         Company.
Swanton, John
1913   Animal Stories from the Indians of the Muskhogean Stock. *Journal
         of American Folklore* 26:193–218.
1915   The Social Significance of the Creek Confederacy. *Proceedings of the
         Nineteenth International Congress of Americanists*, 327–34.
1922   Early History of the Creeks and their Neighbors. *Bureau of American
         Ethnology Bulletin Series* 73.
1928a   Social Organization and Social Usages of the Indians of the Creek
         Confederacy. *Bureau of American Ethnology Annual Report*
         42:23–472.
1928b   Religious Beliefs and Medical Practices of the Creek Indians. *Bureau of
         American Ethnology Annual Report* 42:474–672.
1931   *Modern Square Grounds of the Creek Indians*. Smithsonian Institution,
         Miscellaneous Collections 85(8):1–46.
1932   Introduction to "The Green Corn Dance" by John Howard Payne.
         Chronicles of Oklahoma 10:170–72.
1946   The Indians of the Southeastern United States (repr. 1979). *Bureau of
         American Ethnology Bulletin Series* 137.
Thlopthlocco Tribal Town
1978   *To Keep the Drum, To Tend the Fire: History and Legends of
         Thlopthlocco*. Published for the Thlopthlocco Tribal Town by the
         Oklahoma Indian Affairs Commission.
Timberlake, Henry
1927   *Lieutenant Henry Timberlake's Memoirs*. Edited by Samuel Cole
         Williams. Johnson City, Tenn.: The Watauga Press.
Tuggle, W. O.
1973   *Shem, Ham and Japheth: The Papers of W. O. Tuggle Comprising His
         Indian Diary Sketches and Observations Myths and Washington Journal
         in the Territory and at the Capital, 1879–1882*. Edited by Eugene
         Current-Garcia and Dorothy B. Hatfield. Athens: University of
         Georgia Press.
Vogel, Virgil J.
1990   *American Indian Medicine*. Norman: University of Oklahoma Press.
Waselkov, Gregory A., and Kathryn E. Holland Braund, eds.
1995   *William Bartram on the Southeastern Indians*. Lincoln: University of
         Nebraska Press.
White, Christine Schultz, and Benton R. White
1996   *Now the Wolf Has Come: The Creek Nation in the Civil War*. College
         Station: Texas A&M University Press.
Williams, Samuel Cole
1930   Introduction. In *Adair's History of the American Indians*, edited by Samuel
         Cole Williams, vii–xxix. Johnson City, Tenn.: The Watauga Press.

Woodhouse, S. W.
1992   *A Naturalist in Indian Territory: The Journals of S. W. Woodhouse,*
        1849–1850. Edited by John S. Tomer and Michael J. Brodhead. Norman:
        University of Oklahoma Press.
Woodward, Thomas S
1859   *Woodward's Reminiscences of the Creek, or Muscogee Indians,*
        Contained in Letters to Friends in Georgia and Alabama. Montgomery,
        Ala.: Barrett and Wimbish Book and General Job Printers
        (repr., Tuscaloosa, Ala.: Alabama Book Store, 1939).
Wright, J. Leitch
1986   *Creeks and Seminoles: The Destruction and Regeneration of the*
        Muscogulge People. Lincoln: University of Nebraska Press.
Wyman, William Stokes
1989   Introduction and Notes. In *Creek Indian History: A Historical*
        Narrative of the Genealogy, Traditions and Downfall of the Ispocoga or
        Creek Indian Tribe of Indians, edited by B. V. Pounds. Birmingham, Ala.:
        Birmingham Public Library Press.

INDEX

www.ingramcontent.com/pod-product-compliance
Lightning Source LLC
Chambersburg PA
CBHW022356280326
41935CB00007B/203